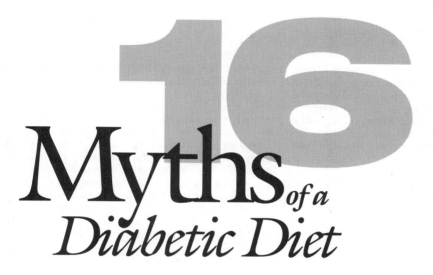

16 Myths *of a* Diabetic Diet

Karen Hanson Chalmers
MS, RD, CDE

Amy E. Peterson
MS, RD, CDE

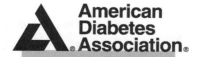
American
Diabetes
Association.

Book Acquisitions, Robert J. Anthony; *Editor,* Aime M. Ballard; *Production Director,* Carolyn R. Segree; *Production Manager,* Peggy M. Rote; *Text Design and Composition,* Harlowe Typography, Inc.; *Cover Design,* Wickham & Associates, Inc.; *Printer,* Transcontinental Printing.

Printed in Canada
1 3 5 7 9 10 8 6 4 2

The suggestions and information contained in this publication are generally consistent with the *Clinical Practice Recommendations* and other policies of the American Diabetes Association, but they do not represent the policy or position of the Association or any of its boards or committees. Reasonable steps have been taken to ensure the accuracy of the information presented. However, the American Diabetes Association cannot ensure the safety or efficacy of any product or service described in this publication. Individuals are advised to consult a physician or other appropriate health care professional before undertaking any diet or exercise program or taking any medication referred to in this publication. Professionals must use and apply their own professional judgment, experience, and training and should not rely solely on the information contained in this publication before prescribing any diet, exercise, or medication. The American Diabetes Association—its officers, directors, employees, volunteers, and members—assumes no responsibility or liability for personal or other injury, loss, or damage that may result from the suggestions or information in this publication.

∞ The paper in this publication meets the requirements of the ANSI Standard Z39.48-1992 (permanence of paper).

ADA titles may be purchased for business or promotional use or for special sales. For information, please write to Lee Romano Sequeira, Special Sales & Promotions, at the address below.

American Diabetes Association
1701 North Beauregard Street
Alexandria, Virginia 22311

Library of Congress Cataloging-in-Publication Data

Chalmers, Karen Hanson.
    16 myths of a "diabetic diet" / Karen Hanson Chalmers, Amy E. Peterson.
        p. cm.
    Includes index.
    ISBN 1-58040-031-0 (pbk. : alk. paper)
        1. Diabetes—Diet therapy. 2. Medical misconceptions. I. Title. II. Title: Sixteen myths of a "diabetic diet." III. Peterson, Amy E., 1964-
RC662 .C45 1999
616.4'620654 21—dc21   99-044966

Dedication

To our patients and Web site friends at the Joslin Clinic,
who have taught us so much about what it means to
live with diabetes

To my supportive and devoted parents, Alden and Flora Hanson,
and my family, with love and respect—KHC

To my parents, Harold and Nancy Peterson, and to Robert Campbell, Jr.,
for all your support, encouragement, and words of wisdom—AEP

To the memory of Raymond Moloney
for his constructive and valuable contributions

Contents

Introduction

People with diabetes have identified "diet" as one of the most difficult parts of managing their disorder. The word diet simply means "the food we eat to nourish our body," and it is important to *all* people. The way you nourish your body affects growth and development, influences how you prevent and fight disease, and dictates your weight, energy level, and how you feel. Unfortunately, over the years, the term diet seems to have taken on a different meaning, particularly for those with diabetes.

The term "diabetic diet" has been around for centuries. One of the earliest references to a diabetic diet is in ancient medical writing dating as far back as 1550 B.C. Today, there are many negative thoughts and feelings associated with the term. However, many positive changes have taken place in nutrition science as it relates to diabetes. From the rigidly controlled, semi-starvation diets prescribed in ancient times, to the "all foods can fit" thinking at the end of the 20th century, we have now arrived at nutrition science as we know it today. The truth now is that there really is no diabetic diet.

When a person is diagnosed with diabetes, their first thoughts and questions usually center on food: "What can I eat?" "What can't I eat?" "How much can I eat?" "Am I always going to be hungry?" "Do I have to give up all of my favorite foods?" "Can I eat pizza and ice cream?" And the list goes on and on. Today, more and more people with diabetes are seeking a registered dietitian's care and counseling so that they may update their knowledge and choose a method of meal planning. Learning about how current research relates to foods and keeping informed of new food products on the market is essential for optimal diabetes management.

Today, one of the most important messages offered by the diabetes team is how to fit diabetes into your lifestyle rather than fitting your lifestyle into your diabetes. An important part of doing that is learning the updated facts about nutrition for your diabetes. This book explores the 16 most common misconceptions about a diabetic diet—the first being that there even is such a thing! Moving beyond these myths is a great step toward better management of your diabetes.

Here's what you'll learn:

- The food that is good for you is the same food that is good for the whole family.
- You do not need a lot of special "diet" foods.
- There are many meal planning options available to obtain optimal diabetes control.
- You can eat a wide choice of foods—variety in meal planning is in!
- Standardized "diabetic diets" are a thing of the past.
- It is no longer necessary to reach an "ideal" weight; moderate weight loss can result in improved control.

Medical Nutrition Therapy Versus the "Diabetic Diet"

Kara: It is so difficult preparing two meals every night—one for me and one for the rest of the family. It's also very expensive.

Dietitian: Why are you preparing two meals? Your eating should not be any different from that of the rest of the family, as long as your family's goal is to eat healthy foods.

Kara: Well, there are so many foods that I can't eat. My neighbor told me I couldn't eat pasta or potatoes, and that bread is a no-no. Everyone knows that fruit is loaded with sugar—and forget the desserts! All those special 'diabetic foods' are so expensive and they aren't as tasty as regular foods.

MYTH:

People with diabetes have to eat different foods from the rest of the family.

Dietitian: The 'diabetic diet' in most people's minds means learning lists of foods they can and cannot eat, restricting sugar, cutting out fat and salt, and eating only a limited amount of starchy foods. That just simply is not how meal planning works today for people with diabetes. With proper education and within the context of healthy eating, a person with diabetes can eat anything a person without diabetes eats. The goals for healthy eating are the same for all Americans: low fat, moderate protein and carbohydrate.

Kara: Do you mean that I can eat the same foods as the rest of my family?

Dietitian: That's right! There are no foods that are 'off limits.' However, some food choices are healthier than others. My job is to simply teach you about healthy eating—and how foods affect your blood glucose.

Kara: When can we get started? I can't wait to start eating like a 'normal' person again.

What's Next?

For many people with and without diabetes, there is much confusion about what to eat. Kara is not alone in thinking that a rigid "diabetic diet" is what is required when you have diabetes. After a couple of visits with her dietitian, Kara learned that there is no diabetic diet; flexible meal planning is what it's all about. The revised diabetes nutrition guidelines make it possible for a person with diabetes to continue to enjoy food and to eat the same foods as the rest of the family. Kara learned that there are no forbidden foods, but rather that some food choices are healthier than others. The decision was hers. What Kara once thought a major challenge is now nothing more than learning how to enjoy favorite foods in a balance with new foods and that *all* foods can be part of a healthy way of eating.

The Old and the New

The diabetes nutrition guidelines of the past were rigid and monotonous. Dietitians had to provide a standardized diabetic diet to all people with diabetes. The diabetic diet was a strict, artificial distribution of calories from carbohydrate, protein, and fat. Patients were told they were expected to reach their "ideal body weight," which was based on height and frame size. The biggest restriction, however, was the strict avoidance of "sugar." Foods with added sugar, such as desserts, were to be strictly avoided. And even the intake of fruit and milk, with their "natural" sugars, was carefully controlled.

The nutrition guidelines of the present are flexible. They offer a wide variety of food choices. Dietitians now recommend that people with diabetes use a meal plan as a guide for healthy eating, with a balance of nutrients tailor-made for each person's food likes and dislikes, lifestyle, health risks, and diabetes medications. Instead of a diabetic diet, meal planning for people with diabetes is now called *medical nutrition therapy*. The recommendations for carbohydrate, protein, and fat are the same as recommendations for all healthy Americans.

Health experts are no longer convinced that achieving so-called ideal body weight should be the primary goal for managing diabetes. Instead, they believe that the goal should be to maintain a reasonable weight—or a weight the patient and the health care provider both feel is realistic and achievable. Even a moderate weight loss of 10–20 pounds for those who are overweight can result in improved blood glucose and blood fat levels.

The goals of medical nutrition therapy are

- To keep blood glucose levels near normal by balancing food with diabetes medications and activity levels.
- To reach optimal levels of fats in the blood (cholesterol and triglycerides).
- To ensure the right amount of calories for keeping or reaching reasonable weight for adults.
- To prevent, delay, or treat food-related risk factors and complications.
- To improve overall health through healthy eating.

Here Are the Facts

The Food Guide Pyramid and the *Dietary Guidelines for Americans*, published by the U.S. Departments of Agriculture and Health and Human Services, provide nutrition guidelines for all healthy Americans and a precise approach to reshape the way Americans eat. They also serve as excellent guides for people with diabetes and their family members. The *Dietary Guidelines for Americans* focuses not only on moderation in what you eat, but also on how excess food relates to America's high rates of obesity, heart disease, high blood pressure, stroke, diabetes, and some forms of cancer. The American diet simply has *too much* fat, cholesterol, and sodium, and *too little* fiber and healthy carbohydrates. Overall health reflects many things, such as environment, heredity, and regular health care, possibly combined with other damaging factors such as smoking, alcohol, and drug use. However, your food choices, which are something you have complete control over, can help you improve your health, based on the following guidelines:

- **Eat a variety of foods.** People with diabetes require the same nutrients, vitamins, and minerals as people without diabetes.
- **Maintain a healthy weight.** Excess body fat makes it harder for people with diabetes to use insulin, which in turn can lead to high blood glucose levels
- **Choose foods low in total fat, saturated fat, and cholesterol.** Diabetes increases the risk for heart and blood vessel disorders.
- **Choose plenty of vegetables, fruits, and grain products.** As well as providing important vitamins and minerals, these foods contain fiber, which can help lower blood fat levels.
- **Eat sweets only in moderation.** High-sugar foods often provide less vitamins, minerals, and fiber, and they tend to be high in fat.
- **If you drink alcoholic beverages, do so in moderation.** Alcohol can affect blood glucose and blood fat levels, as well as supply a lot of empty calories.

The USDA Food Guide Pyramid

The USDA Food Guide Pyramid is a tool that can help you put the above guidelines into effect. It shows what foods Americans eat, what food groups these foods belong in, and how to make the best choices in quantity and quality for good health. You do not have to restrict all foods that are high in fat, cholesterol, and sugar completely. It is your overall intake over time that makes a difference, not a single food or meal. By eating the suggested number of servings, you will ensure that you eat enough fiber and healthy carbohydrates and that you cut down on fat and cholesterol.

The USDA Food Guide Pyramid divides foods into the following groups:

- Level 1 (bottom): Bread, Cereal, Rice, and Pasta Group (6–11 servings)
- Level 2: Vegetable Group (3–5 servings) and Fruit Group (2–4 servings)
- Level 3: Milk, Yogurt, and Cheese Group (2–3 servings) and Meat, Poultry, Fish, Dry Beans, Eggs, and Nuts Group (2–3 servings)
- Level 4: Fats, Oils, and Sweets Group

The Diabetes Food Pyramid

In the Diabetes Food Pyramid, The American Dietetic Association and the American Diabetes Association have made some minor changes to the USDA Food Guide Pyramid to reflect the ways that foods are grouped in meal planning for people with diabetes. For instance, dry beans contain protein, like meats, but they also contain carbohydrates and fiber. The carbohydrates and fiber in beans are more important for diabetes meal planning than the protein. Therefore, in the Diabetes Food Pyramid, beans have been moved to the bottom with other carbo-

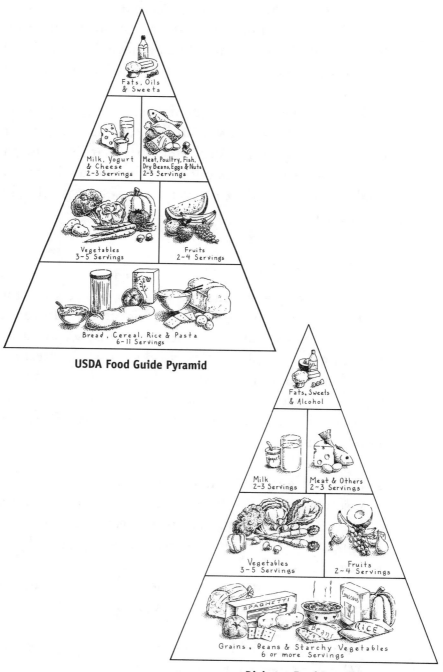

USDA Food Guide Pyramid

Fats, Oils & Sweets

Milk, Yogurt & Cheese 2-3 Servings

Meat, Poultry, Fish, Dry Beans, Eggs & Nuts 2-3 Servings

Vegetables 3-5 Servings

Fruits 2-4 Servings

Bread, Cereal, Rice & Pasta 6-11 Servings

Diabetes Food Pyramid

Fats, Sweets & Alcohol

Milk 2-3 Servings

Meat & Others 2-3 Servings

Vegetables 3-5 Servings

Fruits 2-4 Servings

Grains, Beans & Starchy Vegetables 6 or more Servings

hydrate foods. Another change is that cheese has been moved from the milk group to the meat group. And because the USDA pyramid does not include alcohol, the diabetes pyramid includes it at the top with fats and sweets.

When you use either pyramid, keep in mind that some foods share the same level but have a different number of suggested servings. Also remember that the foods at the bottom level are the ones you should eat the *most*, while the foods at the top level are the ones you should eat the *least*.

Serving Sizes

After looking at the number of suggested servings for each group of foods, it seems like a lot to eat! However, serving sizes are usually smaller than what we are used to seeing on our plate. A portion of food at a restaurant, for example, probably equals more than one "serving." Let's briefly review actual serving sizes of some common foods as grouped according to the Diabetes Food Pyramid:

- Grains, Beans, and Starchy Vegetables:
  1 serving = 1 slice bread, 1/2 cup pasta or potato, 1/2 cup cooked cereal, 1 cup regular cereal, 1/2 cup corn or peas, 1/2 cup lentils or beans, 1 low-fat granola bar
- Vegetables
  1 serving = 1 cup raw vegetables, 1/2 cup cooked vegetables, 1/2 cup vegetable juice
- Fruits
  1 serving = 1 medium piece fresh fruit, 1 cup berries, 1/2 cup canned fruit or juice

- Milk

  1 serving = 1 cup fat-free or low-fat milk, 1 cup fat-free or low-fat yogurt
- Meat and Others

  1 serving = 1 ounce lean fish, meat, or poultry; 1 ounce low-fat cheese, 1 egg
- Fats, Sweets, and Alcohol

  1 serving = 1 teaspoon butter, 1 teaspoon oil, 1 tablespoon salad dressing, 1/2 cup low-fat ice cream, 3 gingersnaps, 1 1/2 ounces liquor, 12 ounces lite beer, 5 ounces wine

Now that you have an idea of serving sizes, it is important to note that you may eat more than one serving in a meal. For example, an acceptable dinner portion of meat (protein) for an active young man might be 5–6 servings (5–6 ounces), while a better dinner portion for an older, less active woman might be 2–3 servings (2–3 ounces). You can determine how many servings you should be eating by working with a registered dietitian who can personalize a meal plan to meet your needs.

Here's What You Can Do

1. Think of yourself as a normal, healthy person who happens to have diabetes. Don't think of your diabetes as a disorder that takes all of the pleasure and taste out of eating. Remember, there are no foods that are off limits.
2. Look at the Diabetes Food Pyramid to find out where most of your calories are coming from. Are you following the pyramid upside down? Are you eating too

much fat and animal products and not enough whole grains, fruits, or vegetables? What do you need to increase? What do you need to decrease?

3. Eat a variety of foods every day from the first three levels of the pyramid.
4. Eat fewer animal products to reduce your risk of heart disease.
5. Eat more fiber by choosing whole-grain breads and cereals. Eat the skins and peels of fresh fruits and vegetables.
6. Eat less fat, especially from foods that contain saturated fats, which are mostly fats that are solid at room temperature.
7. Make a grocery list that includes more of the foods you have been missing. Make an effort to include these foods on a regular basis.
8. If you are trying to lose weight, choose the lower number of suggested servings from each food group. Although the USDA Food Guide Pyramid and Diabetes Food Pyramid were not designed as weight loss tools, they can help you tighten up portion sizes and thereby decrease calories. The lower number of servings will give you about 1,500 calories per day, while the highest number of servings will give you about 2,800 calories per day, which is in the range for a young, active male.
9. Work with your diabetes team and your dietitian to coordinate your food intake with your activity level and diabetes medication(s).
10. Consume meals that contain moderate amounts of protein combined with carbohydrate from starches, fruits, and vegetables. They will satisfy your appetite longer.

11. Educate your family and support system. Help your family members understand how to eat healthfully by achieving variety and balance from all of the food groups.

Commonly Asked Questions

Will I still be able to keep good control of my blood glucose if I eat the same foods as the rest of the family? If you work with your diabetes team and your dietitian to match your food intake with your diabetes medications and activity level, you won't have to eat any differently than the rest of your family, assuming they are eating a healthy, balanced diet.

Why do most people still think that when you have diabetes you have to restrict so many foods? The biggest problem is that many people, with and without diabetes, are not aware that the nutrition guidelines for people with diabetes have changed. Even people with diabetes who have attended nutrition classes or had individual visits with a dietitian may not have received new information since 1994. Some people with many years of diabetes may be strictly avoiding foods that could easily be worked into their meal plan. If you are one of these people, one or two visits with a registered dietitian, preferably one who specializes in diabetes, will get you up to speed. A meeting with a dietitian will show you the opportunities you have to eat just like everyone else—and it will help bring back your enjoyment of food!

Your Turn

Now it's your turn to recall some key points from this chapter. Let's see how you do!

1. Instead of using the term "diabetic diet," we now call meal planning for those with diabetes _____
    _____.

2. Achieving a "reasonable body weight" rather than an "ideal body weight" is now one of the primary goals for diabetes self-management. True or false?

3. Please fill in the number of suggested servings a day from the Diabetes Food Pyramid:

    _____ Grains, Beans, and Starchy Vegetables

    _____ Vegetables

    _____ Fruits

    _____ Milk

    _____ Meat and Others

4. It is your overall food intake over time that makes a difference, not a single food or meal. True or false?

See APPENDIX A for the answers.

2

Sugar

John: I was told last week that I had diabetes! I don't know what to think or do, and my doctor has told me very little except to stay away from sugar and take my medication. Taking my pill is easy, but the eating part is hard. What do I eat?

Dietitian: You must be feeling completely overwhelmed with your new diagnosis and very little nutrition education. The main goal of medical nutrition therapy for diabetes is not to avoid sugar, but to eat a healthy balance of foods spread out over the day.

John: But I thought people with diabetes couldn't eat sugar because it makes the blood sugar go up too high and too fast.

MYTH:

People with diabetes can eat as much as they want as long as the food does not contain sugar.

Dietitian: Actually, the new nutrition guidelines that the American Diabetes Association published in 1994 state that sugar is *just a carbohydrate* and that it can be added into any healthy eating plan in moderation.

What's Next?

The idea that it's necessary to avoid sugar is one of the biggest misconceptions in diabetes management today. Like John, many people with diabetes mistakenly believe that they must work very hard to eliminate *all* foods with sugar. But no one can avoid sugar completely. It would be an almost impossible task because many healthy foods contain some form of sugar. Some sugar is added, and some is found naturally in foods. Many research studies completed over the past 20 years have demonstrated that foods containing sugar can be part of a healthy diet, even for people with diabetes, and that dental cavities are the only health risk linked to a moderate intake of sugar. After a couple of meetings with the dietitian, John learned that sugar is not forbidden or harmful, and he began to feel comfortable fitting many new foods into his food plan.

The Old and the New

Nutrition therapy has always been the cornerstone in the self-management of diabetes. Followers of Hippocrates, a physician in ancient Greece, promoted a diet with large amounts of carbohydrate to replace sugar lost in the urine of those with diabetes, in combination with opium, which was used as an appetite suppressant. By the sixth century, diabetes was attributed to eating an excessive amount of food with sugar and flour; therefore, many carbohydrate foods were eliminated from the diet of people with diabetes. From that time until insulin was discovered in 1921, the carbohydrate intake of a person with diabetes only consisted of vegetables such as onions, lettuce, radishes, cabbage, and mustard greens.

Finally, after many years of diabetes research, insulin was isolated in 1921. The "starvation diet" approach to treating diabetes took a giant step backward, while liberalized and nutritious food choices started taking baby steps forward. Although fruits were still mostly restricted at that time, carbohydrate intake was on the upswing. The amount of carbohydrate recommended for people with diabetes has increased from 20% of calories in 1921 to what the American Diabetes Association now recommends. The number of calories from carbohydrate is now based on an individual's blood glucose (blood sugar), weight, and lipid levels (up to 55–60% of calories). However, it wasn't until the 1980s, when self-monitoring of blood glucose was introduced, that health professionals started to understand how certain carbohydrates really affect blood glucose levels.

For years, people with diabetes were taught to avoid *concentrated sweets*, known as *simple sugars*, because they were thought to overload the blood with glucose much faster than *starches*, which are known as *complex carbohydrates*. Dr. Elliott Joslin stated the general consensus about starch and sugar best in his early editions of *Joslin's Diabetic Manual for Doctor and Patient*:

> Sugar enters the blood as fast as a child runs
> Starch enters the blood as fast as a child walks
> Starch in vegetables enters the blood as slowly as a child creeps

This explanation was used when emphasizing to people with diabetes how important it was to avoid sugar strictly, measure starchy foods carefully, and to eat vegetables more freely.

We followed the assumption that sugar was harmful to people with diabetes until the 1970s, when scientists started to look for clear evidence of how sugar and diabetes interacted. The American Diabetes Association and prominent researchers in the field of diabetes studied the published findings from many scientific studies on nutrition and diabetes for many years. They concluded in the *Nutrition Principles for the Management of Diabetes and Related Complications, 1994*, that there was little scientific evidence to suggest that sugar is more quickly digested and absorbed into the bloodstream than starch or that sugar elevates blood glucose more than starch. Sugar, we have learned, has about the same effect on blood glucose as any other carbohydrate. Therefore, the use of sugar (sucrose) as part of the *total* carbohydrate content of the diet is okay for people with diabetes as long as these sugar-containing foods are substituted for other carbohydrate foods as part of a balanced meal plan. Nutrition therapy is not about *avoiding* sugar but rather about controlling blood glucose.

What Is Sugar?

The three types of carbohydrate are *sugars, starches,* and *fibers.* These carbohydrates are all made up of a certain number of "sugar blocks." Sugar blocks may be single blocks, double blocks, or many blocks connected together in long chains. All carbohydrates have about the same number of calories. Carbohydrates do, however, vary in their chemical structure and in the number of units, or sugar blocks, that are put together to make them. Sugars are made up of only one or two sugar blocks and are called *simple carbohydrates.* Starches and fibers are made up of many sugar blocks connected together and are called *complex carbohydrates.*

There are six important sugars in nutrition. Three are *single* sugars (*mono*saccharides), and three are *double* sugars (*di*saccharides), which are made up of pairs of single sugars. The single sugar blocks (monosaccharides) are

- Glucose
- Fructose
- Galactose

The double sugar blocks (disaccharides) are

- Maltose (glucose + glucose)
- Sucrose (glucose + fructose)
- Lactose (glucose + galactose)

Starch and fiber are called *poly*saccharides and are composed of straight or branched chains of the single sugar blocks. In this chapter, we're mostly talking about sugars, or simple carbohydrates, because those are the carbohydrates that many people with diabetes think they have to avoid. See chapter 3 for more information about starches and fibers.

The Monosaccharides

Glucose is the largest, the most common, and the most complicated of all of the sugars. Glucose is always found as one of the two sugars in disaccharides. It is also the basic unit of starch and fiber. When carbohydrates are digested, they are converted into glucose, which our bodies use for fuel, and our blood glucose (sugar) levels rise. Almost 100% of carbohydrate foods break down into glucose.

Fructose is the sweetest of the sugars and makes up table sugar (sucrose) in combination with glucose. Fructose occurs naturally in fruits, berries, vegetables, and honey. It is also used as an additive in products sweetened with high-fructose corn syrup. Although many people with diabetes believe fructose may be a better choice as a sweetener than sucrose, the American Diabetes Association states that "fructose may have no overall advantage as a sweetening agent."

Galactose is not as common as glucose or fructose, and it does not occur freely in nature. It is one of the three monosaccharides common in foods, but its sugar block is always connected to another sugar block (glucose) to form lactose, the sugar in milk.

The Disaccharides

Maltose consists of two glucose units and is a part of only a few foods. Maltose appears when starch is broken down, such as when food is digested, when seeds germinate, and when alcohol is fermented.

Sucrose consists of fructose and glucose and forms what we know as table sugar. It is the most common of all the sugars and gets its sweet taste from fructose. The main food sources of sucrose are the juices from sugar cane and sugar beets. These juices are processed to make brown, white, or powdered sugar. Today, sucrose can be part of an eating plan for *anyone* with diabetes. It is no longer forbidden or restricted, although it should be used in moderation.

Lactose, which consists of galactose and glucose, is found in the milk of mammals. Lactose is the main carbohydrate found in milk, and it is often referred to as milk sugar.

Where Is It Found?

Natural or Added?

So now you know that a sugar—any kind of sugar—is just a carbohydrate, that sucrose (table sugar) is only one type of sugar among several that are found in foods, and that a sugar has about the same effect on blood glucose as any other carbohydrate. However, you still need to think about how sugars occur in food: Does the food contain sugar *naturally,* or has sugar been *added*? Natural or added sugars may have the same effect on blood glucose, but the foods that contain these sugars may not be equally healthy or nutritious.

For instance, an orange contains carbohydrate in the form of the natural sugar called fructose, while a candy bar contains its carbohydrate from the added sugar called sucrose. We all know the orange is healthier because it is a good source of many vitamins, minerals, and fiber. The candy bar, on the other hand, is what we call an *empty-calorie food,* which means that while it may taste good, it doesn't offer any health benefits. The candy bar also contributes a great deal of fat and calories. If you occasionally choose to eat an empty-calorie food, your body does not see any difference between the natural or added sugars when it comes to blood glucose. However, you will need to substitute that food for another carbohydrate food at that time because your blood glucose will react to the total amount of carbohydrate you have eaten. A dietitian can help you learn how you can safely include the occasional empty-calorie food in your meal plan.

Finding the Sugar

One way to find sugar in foods is to look at the food label. In the nutrition facts section, look under the "sugar" category. If you look in the ingredient list, the sugars in the product will be listed individually, but they're often listed under names that most consumers do not recognize as sugars. The following list gives just some of the obvious and less obvious sugar names to look for: brown sugar, confectionery sugar, carob, corn syrup, dextrose, fructose, galactose, glucose, honey, invert sugar, lactose, maltose, maple syrup, molasses, sucrose, and turbinado.

Some sugars listed in the ingredient list but not necessarily in the nutrition facts section include the sugar alcohols: hydrogenated starch hydrolysate, sorbitol, mannitol, maltitol, isomalt, and xylitol. The manufacturer is not required to include these sugar alcohols as part of the sugar grams on a food label unless the food is called *sugar free*. Sugar alcohols may be listed as "other" or as "sugar alcohols" directly under the category "sugars," or they may be found only in the ingredient list. However, *all* sugars have to be added into the total carbohydrate grams. So overall, it is more important to look at the total carbohydrate grams than at the sugar grams.

Why Do We Need It?

We don't really need sugar; however, sugar is found in many healthy foods and it tastes good. Natural sugars, such as those found in fruits, vegetables, and milk make up about half of the sugar intake in the United States. Added sugars, such as those found in cookies, soda, cakes, and candy, make up the other half of our sugar intake.

The Upside and Downside of Sugar

Sugar has received bad reviews for many years. Aside from the sweet taste that sugar adds to food, the only proven information that we have about sugar is that it contributes to tooth decay if eaten in excessive amounts. But we also know that if eaten in moderation, sugar is not necessarily harmful to our health. Let's clear up some of the confusion about sugar by looking at the upside and the downside of this controversial carbohydrate.

The Downside

1. **Extra calories:** Many empty-calorie foods, such as candy, cake, and ice cream, give you fuel and pleasure, but without the benefit of vitamins, minerals, fiber, and protein. If you are eating 15–20 grams of carbohydrate in the form of a candy bar instead of a piece of fruit, not only will you be taking in more calories (from fat), but you will also be giving up a healthy food for a not-so-healthy food. Even the "fat-free" versions of many of these empty-calorie foods will give you extra calories because the maker has to add more carbohydrate (sugar and/or starch) to stabilize the product when the fat is taken out. Dessert foods should not replace healthier foods on a regular basis, whether you have diabetes or not.

2. **Small portion sizes:** Often if you eat a food that gets a lot of its total carbohydrate content from sugar (sucrose), you'll have to eat a smaller quantity. For example, 1 cup of Cheerios contains about **19 grams** of total carbohydrate:

   1 gram coming from sugar
   2 grams coming from fiber
   16 grams coming from starch

   However, 1 cup of Frosted Cheerios contains **26 grams** of total carbohydrate:

   14 grams coming from sugar
   1 gram coming from fiber
   11 grams coming from starch

   Let's say that your meal plan allows you to eat 30 grams of carbohydrate from cereal for breakfast. You could eat about 1 3/4 cups of regular Cheerios, but you'd only be able to eat 1 1/4 cups of the Frosted Cheerios. You can leave it up to your appetite to decide which one you want.

3. **Dental caries (cavities):** The digestive process begins in the mouth as soon as we start chewing food. Both sugar and starch break down into glucose in the mouth and contribute equally to tooth decay. Bacteria in the mouth thrive on food and ferment the sugars in carbohydrate foods. During the fermentation process, the bacteria produce and leave behind an acid that eats away at tooth enamel, causing dental caries, or cavities. The whole decaying process actually depends on how long the food stays in the mouth. However, regular brushing and flossing along with limiting large amounts of sticky carbohydrate foods will help prevent cavities.

The Upside

1. **Sugar does not cause health problems** such as obesity, hyperactivity in adults and children, diabetes, or heart disease when eaten in moderation. Although sugar may contribute to weight gain and obesity if eaten in excessive amounts, it has actually been documented that obese people eat less sugar than do thin people. And although excessive levels of sugar can affect blood lipids (fats), which in turn promotes heart disease, moderate sugar intake does not increase the risk of heart disease.
2. **Sugar is useful as a food additive** to enhance and balance flavor and to supply color and texture (that

brown, crusty texture in baked goods). Sugar also acts as a preservative by balancing and binding moisture, which keeps foods "fresh." It adds bulk to ice cream and baked goods, helps to retain air in light-textured products, balances acidity, and lowers the freezing point of foods.

Here's What You Can Do

1. **Use sugar as part of your *total* carbohydrate intake.** This does not mean you should eat unlimited amounts of sugar or dessert foods, but rather eat these foods in *moderation*. Totally eliminating sugar is unnecessary and impossible.
2. **Use less of all sugars and dessert foods,** whether you have diabetes or not.
3. **Read food labels** to determine how much of the carbohydrate is coming from sugar and if the food is nutritious rather than just an empty-calorie food.
4. **If you eat a high-sugar food, use the serving size as your guide.** Most average-size cookies list one to two cookies as a serving size, while ice creams list 1/2 cup as a serving size. Most people eat at least twice as much, especially ice cream!
5. **Be sensible, but enjoy your new food choices.** It is not "cheating" to eat foods that have sugar in them as long as your meals are within the context of healthy eating. You are not a bad person for enjoying *all* foods. You are a normal person who happens to have diabetes, living in the real world.

Summary

It has been more than 5 years since the American Diabetes Association published the *Nutrition Principles for the Management of Diabetes and Related Complications*, yet people with diabetes still believe avoiding sugar is the main goal of nutrition therapy. After years of educating people with diabetes about the dangers of sugar and giving them lists of "good" and "bad" foods, we now know that sugar is just a carbohydrate and that it has about the same effect on blood glucose as any other carbohydrate. The guidelines for sugar apply not only to those with diabetes, but rather to *all* healthy Americans. With the proper education from a registered dietitian, you can learn how to choose your carbohydrates wisely.

Your Turn

Now it's your turn to recall some key points from this chapter. Let's see how you do!

1. One of the biggest misconceptions in diabetes self-management today is that people with diabetes must avoid _____.
2. There is *little* scientific evidence to suggest that sugar is more quickly digested and absorbed into the bloodstream or that sugar elevates blood sugar more than starch. True or false?
3. The three types of carbohydrate are _____, _____, and _____.

4. _____, _____, and _____ are the three food groups that make up about half of the natural sugar intake in the United States.
5. Two examples of empty-calorie foods are _____ and _____.
6. Using foods with added sugar as part of your total carbohydrate content should be done in moderation. True or false?

See APPENDIX A for the answers.

3

Starch and Fiber

Jan: I know what fiber is, but aren't the foods that are high in fiber also high in carbohydrate? I love brown rice, whole-grain breads, and all sorts of beans, but do you know how much carbohydrate these foods contain? I want to increase the fiber in my diet, but it's hard to eat fiber foods without eating too much carbohydrate. Why does the American Diabetes Association recommend starches?

Dietitian: Starches and fiber are recommended not only by the American Diabetes Association, but also by the American Dietetic Association. And they're recommended for *all* people. When you look at the USDA Food Guide Pyramid, you will notice that the foods

MYTH:

People with diabetes should not eat too many starchy foods, even if they contain fiber, because starch raises your blood glucose and makes you gain weight.

27

containing the most starch and fiber are located in the bottom two levels of the pyramid. This means they should be the most abundant foods on your plate.

Jan: But I heard that all carbohydrates, particularly starches, make you *gain* weight and are the main *cause* of diabetes—not sugar! Should I cut out all of the starchy foods like potatoes, beans, pasta, rice, and wheat and then substitute these foods with foods like raw vegetables and salad to get enough fiber?

Dietitian: Starches and sugar do not cause diabetes or weight gain. Starch, sugar, and fiber are all types of carbohydrate. Carbohydrates are our body's main source of fuel, and we need them. Unfortunately, many Americans eat excessive amounts of carbohydrate because they are not looking at the carbohydrate content of the foods they eat. Bread, rice, and beans are just some examples of foods that have carbohydrate coming from starch and fiber. The carbohydrate from these foods can add up very quickly at a meal, especially when added to other carbohydrate foods at the same meal. However, these same foods also provide natural sources of fiber, and it is important to eat these foods daily.

Jan: So if you eat too much in quantity, it can make you gain weight and raise your blood glucose?

Dietitian: Right. It isn't the starches or the sugars themselves—it's the quantity!

What's Next?

Many people view starchy foods as "bad" foods and try to eliminate many of these foods from their daily intake.

When these same people also think of sugary foods as bad foods, they end up eliminating many healthy food choices (carbohydrates), as well as good sources of fiber, vitamins, and minerals. Jan learned from the dietitian that starch and sugar are just two of the three types of carbohydrate that belong in everyone's eating plan. Jan also learned that many carbohydrate foods also contain the third type of carbohydrate called fiber, which she was attempting to increase to make her feel more satisfied and full after eating a meal, without adding extra calories.

Jan's dietitian taught her how to keep track of her starch and sugar intake with a meal planning method called carbohydrate counting. (See chapter 7.) This meal planning method gave Jan a "carbohydrate allowance" to spend at each meal and snack. Much to her surprise, Jan was able to incorporate many new and different foods into her meals and snacks. Jan learned that it doesn't matter where the carbohydrate is coming from (starch or sugar) but rather how much total carbohydrate you are eating at each meal and snack: *a carbohydrate is a carbohydrate*. By monitor-ing how much carbohydrate she was eating throughout the day, Jan was able to improve her blood glucose levels. She also found it easier to control her weight by adding fiber-rich foods that helped her feel full and satisfied. Jan now is more comfortable eating the foods she likes.

The Old and the New

Before insulin was discovered in 1921, rigid restriction of carbohydrate intake was the only means of controlling blood glucose. People with diabetes were told not to eat sugar or starch. And they were allowed only a small amount of fiber from certain foods. Vegetable foods were divided into categories based on their carbohydrate contents. The first category, 3% vegetables, included lettuce, cucumbers, spinach, asparagus, celery, and cabbage. These were allowed in unlimited quantities. The second category, 6% vegetables, included pumpkin, turnip, squash, beets, carrots, onions, and very young, fresh peas. The third category, 15% vegetables, included mature peas, lima beans, and parsnips. The foods in the fourth and last category, 20% vegetables, were to be used only with caution. These starchy foods, such as potatoes, corn, bread, rice, macaroni, and beans, were only allowed in very small quantities and had to be carefully measured.

With the discovery of insulin, the amount of carbohydrate allowed in the form of starch was gradually increased to about 20% of the total daily calories, although sugar in most forms, including many fruits, was still forbidden. As research has advanced to show that starch and sugar have similar effects on blood glucose and that a diet high in fat is related to heart disease, the recommended percentage of daily calories from carbohydrate has increased, while the recommended percentage of daily calories from fat has decreased. Today, all people, including people with diabetes, are encouraged to eat a liberal amount of carbohydrate, including starch and fiber. A registered dietitian can help people with diabetes determine how much they should eat based on factors such as blood glucose control, weight, and lipid levels.

What Are Starch and Fiber?

As we learned in chapter 3, starch and fiber are commonly known as *complex carbohydrates*. Starch and fiber are only found in plants, and their structure is composed of straight or branched chains of 10 or more sugar-blocks called *polysaccharides*. Like other carbohydrates, when we eat starch, it is converted into glucose, which we use for fuel. Because starch is made up of many sugar-blocks bonded together, these sugar-blocks have to be broken down into their components before they can be used. The cooking, chewing, and digestive process breaks the bonds holding the sugar-blocks together. Within a couple of hours after eating, all the starch is usually digested and its glucose is being used as fuel by the cells of the body. The best sources of starch are the grains, such as rice, wheat, corn, millet, rye, barley, and oats. Legumes (plants of the bean and pea family) and tubers, such as potatoes and yams, also provide starch.

Fiber is the "roughage" that comes from plant foods that cannot be digested by the human digestive system. It is considered the *nonstarch polysaccharide* and is made up of cellulose, hemicellulose, pectins, gums, mucilages, and lignins. Fiber is what gives plants their structure, and it is found in all plant foods, such as vegetables, fruits, grains, and legumes. Fiber also adds bulk that helps push foods through your digestive tract. Unlike the other two carbohydrates, sugar and starch, fiber cannot be broken down into glucose for fuel because we do not have the enzymes, or "helpers," needed to break the bonds that hold its sugar-blocks together. Although there is some energy available from indigestible carbohydrate, fiber gives us very limited amounts of fuel and calories.

Where Are Starch and Fiber Found?

Starch

The base of the USDA Food Guide Pyramid (see chapter 1) features foods rich in starch and fiber. This group includes breads, cereals, rice and pasta, dry beans, and starchy vegetables. The healthiest choices of breads and cereals are those made from whole grains, which means that the whole kernel of grain is left in the flour used to make them. White flour has the bran (coarse outer layer) removed from the kernel of grain to give a lighter texture. Some specific foods in this category are listed below to give you an idea of how much one serving is:

Breads, Cereals, Rice, Pasta, Starchy Vegetables
(15 grams of carbohydrate each)

1 slice of bread	1/2 cup pasta, potato, corn,
1/2 English muffin or small bagel	green peas
3/4 cup dry cereal or 1/2 cup	3 Tbsp. flour
hot cereal	4–6 crackers
1/3 cup rice, beans, lentils	3 cups popcorn

Fiber

Fiber is classified as either *soluble* or *insoluble*. Both soluble and insoluble fibers in food are called *dietary fiber*. Soluble fiber absorbs water. It is found in citrus fruits, apples, strawberries, vegetables, oat and rice bran, barley, and dried beans and peas (legumes). This fiber cannot retain its structure in the digestion process and becomes gummy. A gel is formed when it is mixed with water. Soluble fiber slows the process of food emptying from the stomach. Insoluble fiber does not absorb water. This fiber is able to retain its structure in the digestion process and is known as roughage. Insoluble fiber is found in wheat and corn bran, whole grains, and mature fruits and vegetables, particularly root vegetables. The amount of insoluble fiber in a food can be subtracted from the total carbohydrate to determine the amount of *available carbohydrate*.

Why Do We Need Starch and Fiber?

Foods that contain complex carbohydrates, such as grains, breads, cereal, rice, pasta, fruits, vegetables, and legumes, are healthy sources of fuel. Although sugar (simple carbohydrates) is also a source of fuel, it should be eaten in moderation. Dessert-type foods that are high in sugar do not provide fiber, may contain a lot of fat, and are often limited in nutrition. However, foods such as fruits, vegetables, and milk contain many nutrients, as well as forms of sugar, and are healthy sources of fuel. Some foods contain both simple and complex carbohydrates. For example, fruits and vegetables contain both sugar and fiber. Most starches, as well as fruits, vegetables, and legumes, are low in fat, high in fiber, and contain nutrients such as vitamins A, B complex, C, and E; beta carotene; folic acid; zinc; iron; calcium; and selenium. The bulk of our diet, whether we have diabetes or not, should come from foods that are high in complex carbohydrates.

The Upside and the Downside of Starch and Fiber

The good news for people with diabetes is that *all* carbohydrate foods, including starches and fibers, can fit into a healthy way of eating. The body breaks down all carbohydrate, except fiber, into glucose (blood sugar) at the same rate, although this may be influenced by factors such as cooking method and the presence of fat and protein in the same meal. Therefore, first and foremost, it is important to control the total amount of carbohydrate eaten.

The Downside

1. Eating a lot of carbohydrate from starch can lead to weight gain. Excess calories from *any* food will be stored as body fat.
2. Starchy foods, such as cake, cookies, muffins, sweet breads, and cereals, have higher amounts of total carbohydrate because of the starch *plus* the added sugar. Even though these foods may be part of a healthy diet, they may lead to higher blood glucose levels and to weight gain. Therefore, the portion sizes should be carefully monitored.
3. If taken in excessive amounts, even fiber may be harmful. If a lot of fiber is consumed in a short period of time, it can cause intestinal gas, bloating, cramps, and impaction. Eating too much fiber, which attracts water, could lead to dehydration. When you increase the amount of fiber in your diet, you should also increased the amount of water you drink to 6–8 cups per day. Fiber in very large amounts can also interfere

in the absorption of some minerals, such as zinc, iron, magnesium, and calcium.

The Upside

1. Whole-grain, high-fiber foods tend to be low in fat and calories (fiber does not provide calories or fuel) and can often replace or prevent you from eating too much fat and protein from animal products. This can reduce your risk for heart disease and high blood glucose.
2. Whole-grain, high-fiber foods make you feel full and satisfied at meals and snacks, without adding extra calories. They help to prevent overeating or going back for an extra helping. These foods also take longer to chew, so your brain has adequate time to notify your stomach that you are full.
3. Whole-grain, high-fiber foods form a large bulk in the intestine and help push the food through the digestive tract at a faster rate. This results in less pressure on the walls of the intestine, thereby reducing the risk of problems such as constipation and hemorrhoids.
4. Many studies have positively linked soluble fiber intake to lowering the risk of heart disease by reducing total blood cholesterol.

Here's What You Can Do

1. A healthy fiber intake is between 20 and 35 grams each day. To eat this amount, many Americans would have to *double* their intake.

2. Eat a variety of carbohydrate foods to ensure that you get the health benefits from soluble and insoluble fiber.
3. Eat 3 or more servings of vegetables each day: 1 serving equals 1/2 cup cooked or 1 cup raw vegetables.
4. Eat 2 or more servings of fruit each day: 1 serving equals 1 small to medium-sized piece of fruit or 1/2 cup canned or 1 cup cut-up fresh fruit.
5. Eat at least 6 servings of grain products or legumes a day: 1 serving equals 1 slice of whole-grain bread, 1/2 cup of brown rice or pasta, 1 small potato with the skin, or 1/2 cup of legumes.
6. Eat fewer processed foods. Make sure the first ingredient listed on the label of breads, cereals, crackers, etc. is a whole-grain flour (for example, whole-wheat flour instead of just wheat flour). Note that "whole-wheat bread" is *not* the same as "wheat bread."
7. Use low-fat, low-calorie toppings on starchy foods instead of the high-fat toppings that add too many calories (for example, try using salsa on your baked potato instead of sour cream).
8. To get the fiber, leave the skin and peels on fruits and vegetables, if possible. Fruits with seeds, such as raspberries and strawberries, also contain a lot of fiber.
9. Use whole-grain flours when cooking and baking.
10. Check with your doctor or dietitian before taking a fiber pill or supplement. Fiber replacements lack other nutrients found in actual fiber-containing foods.

Summary

For years, starch has been thought of as the fattening part of foods. Don't forget, however, that many starchy foods are eaten with added fat! When we eat potatoes, bread, corn, pasta, or vegetables, we rarely eat them without putting some sort of fat on top, such as butter, margarine, sour cream, cream cheese, or cheese sauce. What about a pasta meal? Not only are we served large quantities of pasta, but we also add several slices of Italian bread, breaded cutlets, and perhaps croutons on the salad, most of which contain carbohydrate in the form of starch. By the end of the meal, the carbohydrate has added up to an excessive amount. It isn't the starch or the pasta that causes weight gain and high blood glucose, it's the *total amount of calories from carbohydrate* that is consumed, along with the *fat and protein.*

Three things provide fuel to the human body: carbohydrate, protein, and fat. Protein foods provide the most expensive fuel, take longer to empty from the stomach, and do not provide the quantity of fuel that carbohydrate does. Because most Americans already eat too much protein and too many animal products, which put us at high risk for heart disease, many can ill afford to add more, financially or healthwise. The fuel from fatty foods is not used efficiently by the brain and the central nervous system. Fat also provides twice as many calories as carbohydrate and protein, and it is linked to overweight and obesity if consumed in large amounts. So that leaves us with carbohydrate as the major fuel source for our body. Food starch is probably the most important fuel source for energy and the fuel most preferred by our brains and nervous systems.

Contrary to what you hear from the promoters of the many low-carbohydrate "diets" now on the market, the healthiest diet recommended by health professionals and the USDA is the one depicted in the food pyramid. Promoters of low-carbohydrate diets dismiss evidence offered by well-known researchers and proven studies, and they condemn carbohydrate as the culprit that causes diabetes, high blood glucose, and weight gain. However, the Food Guide Pyramid actually directs Americans on how to eat in a balanced and healthy way by eating plenty of carbohydrate- and fiber-rich foods, moderate amounts of protein, and low amounts of fat.

Your Turn

Now it's your turn to recall some key points from this chapter. Let's see how you do!

1. Fiber is only found in plant foods. True or false?
2. The only one of the three carbohydrates that will *not* give us much fuel for energy but does help us to feel full and satisfied after a meal is _____.
3. The base, or foundation, of the USDA Food Guide Pyramid features foods rich in _____ and _____.
4. Food starch is the most important and preferred source of fuel for our brain and nervous system. True or false?

See APPENDIX A for the answers.

4

Protein

Mark: I've been reading that it's important to eat a high-protein, low-carbohydrate diet to help keep my blood sugars down.

Dietitian: While it is important to get an adequate amount of protein in our diets, most of us get too much. We still need to obtain most of our calories from carbohydrate rather than protein, even with diabetes, because our bodies use carbohydrate for energy.

Mark: Okay, but since I'm exercising more to lose weight, shouldn't I be eating a lot of protein or even taking protein supplements to build more muscle?

Dietitian: No. The only way to build stronger muscles is with regular exercise

MYTH:

People with diabetes should eat a lot of protein to stay healthy and strong.

39

and a balanced meal plan that contains most of its calories in carbohydrate, not protein. Too much protein may even be harmful to your kidneys.

What's Next?

Like Mark, most people think they don't eat enough protein. There have been so many misconceptions over the years about protein and what it can do for us that we sometimes wonder if we truly get enough. People with diabetes often end up eating more protein and less carbohydrate in an effort to control blood glucose levels. And if you're looking to "bulk up," you may be considering trying out those cans of protein powders in the health food stores (after all, muscles are made of protein, so it makes sense to eat more protein to build bigger muscles, right?). Unfortunately, most of us eat too much protein, often at the expense of other nutrients. This can potentially lead to some serious health problems. Let's take a look at the truth behind some of these misconceptions about protein.

The Old and the New

The history of the role of protein in the diets of people with diabetes has been long and ever changing. Before the discovery of insulin, the only course of treatment for diabetes involved dietary measures. Because people with diabetes were extremely limited in the amount of carbohydrate they could eat, the prescribed diets were usually high in protein and/or fat—and often involved eating very strange foods, such as suet, blood, and even 10 to 40 egg yolks every day!

In the early 1900s, Dr. Elliot Joslin recommended limiting protein intake to 1 gram per kilogram of body weight because too much protein in the diet was found to increase both nitrogen and glucose in the urine, further aggravating diabetes. Have you ever been told that approximately 50–60% of the protein that you eat gets converted into blood glucose? This information came about in the 1930s using eggs, casein (a milk protein), and meat in studies of how protein affects metabolism in people with diabetes. We still use this information today, although some recent studies have challenged whether this "fact" is indeed true.

Much has changed over the years regarding the best "diet" for someone with diabetes. Because there are only three main nutrients to work with, diets have ranged from high fat to high protein to high carbohydrate. Even today, with some of the most advanced treatments for diabetes ever, leading health and diabetes authorities still can't decide which is the best diet for diabetes. Some believe a higher-protein diet is best, while others argue that a diet high in complex carbohydrates is the way to go, since a higher-protein diet may bring an increased risk for kidney problems down the road. Who is right? We may not have a definitive answer right now, but read on to learn more about this controversial nutrient, protein.

What Is Protein?

The word protein comes from the Greek word *proteios*, which means "of the first rank." No wonder we give it such importance in our diets! A protein is an organic substance made up of carbon, hydrogen, and oxygen (just like carbohydrate). Unlike carbohydrate, however, protein also contains nitrogen. These atoms are arranged into amino acids, which then are linked into chains to form protein molecules. Amino acids are the building blocks of proteins, and there are 22 amino acids that are linked together in various combinations to form different types of protein molecules. Nine of these amino acids are called "essential" because our bodies cannot make them; they must be obtained from foods that we eat. It is important that we eat foods that contain essential amino acids because our cells need all 22 amino acids to make body proteins.

Why Do We Need Protein?

Protein has many important functions in the body. These include:

- creating new cells when old ones die
- forming antibodies (which fight viruses and bacteria)
- creating visual pigment to help us see
- forming enzymes (for example, digestive enzymes)
- forming certain hormones (such as insulin)

All of the cells in our bodies contain protein. In fact, approximately 50% of the body's weight comes from protein. Our hair, nails, muscles, cartilage, bones, and body fluids contain many different kinds of protein.

When we eat foods that contain protein, the protein is digested into its building blocks, the amino acids. Our bodies make a decision as to how those amino acids will be used and then arrange amino acids in a specific order, based on what types of proteins are needed. For example, the protein needed to help blood to clot (called thrombin) will have a different sequence of amino acids than the kind of protein needed to make insulin. Whatever amino acids are "left over" from protein synthesis will be stored as—you guessed right—fat.

How Much Protein Do We Need?

Most people in the U.S. grow up believing that a meal isn't a meal unless protein is present, usually in the form of a piece of steak, a hamburger, or perhaps a chicken breast. After all, who could stay healthy just by eating a plate of spaghetti? Surprisingly, although we do need to eat some protein every day, we need much less than you may think. On average, people in the U.S. consume approximately 15% of their calories from protein, which translates into 1.5 grams of protein per kilogram of body weight. This is *twice* what is needed to meet our daily requirements, whether we have diabetes or not.

The recommended dietary allowance (RDA) for protein is 0.8 grams per kilogram of body weight for adults. (We actually need only 0.6 grams of protein per kilogram of body weight to stay healthy, but a margin of safety is built into the RDA.) To give you an example, a man who weighs 170 pounds (77 kilograms) needs 62 grams of protein in his diet every day. A woman who weighs 130 pounds (59 kilograms) only needs 47 grams per day. Infants, children, and adolescents require more protein for growth and development; therefore, the RDAs are higher (0.9–2.2 grams per kilogram of body weight per day). Protein needs are increased during pregnancy and lactation, as well.

Diabetes and Protein Requirements

There is no longer a set "diabetic diet" for people with diabetes, but it is recommended that between 10 and 20% of total calories come from protein, with the majority of calories coming from carbohydrate and the remainder from fat. There is no evidence that a higher or lower intake of protein is beneficial for blood glucose control. In other words, the RDAs for protein apply to people with diabetes as well as to people without diabetes.

More recently, however, some studies have shown that people with type 2 diabetes may actually benefit from a slightly higher protein intake. The "theory" that approximately 50–60% of protein in food gets converted to blood glucose (dating back to the early part of this century) has been challenged. A few studies have shown that blood glucose levels do not rise in people with type 2 diabetes fed a diet containing a moderate amount of protein. Perhaps not as much protein is metabolized into glucose as we once thought. A similar effect has been seen in people with type 1 diabetes, although *large* amounts of protein ingested do require more insulin to prevent high blood glucose levels.

Does this mean that if you have type 2 diabetes, you can eat more protein in your diet without it affecting your diabetes control? It's probably too soon to make any conclusions. The best way for you to determine how protein affects *your* blood glucose control, whether at a meal or at a snack is to check your blood glucose after you eat. It's also important not to eat too much protein because extra protein intake means extra calories. And there is a risk of too much protein leading to—or worsening—kidney damage, as well as leading to other diseases, such as heart disease, some types of cancer, and osteoporosis.

Where Is Protein Found?

Once you know how much protein you need every day, you need to learn what foods contain protein. However, you most likely know this already! Chances are, you are picturing steak, pork chops, turkey, and fish. *Animal sources* of protein include red meats (beef, pork, lamb, veal), poultry (chicken, turkey, duck, goose), seafood (fish, shellfish), and dairy foods (milk, yogurt, cheese, eggs). These animal protein foods contain all of the

TABLE 1: Protein Content of Some Animal Foods

Food (4 ounces, cooked, unless noted)	Protein (grams)
Chicken breast, skinless	35
Turkey breast, skinless	33
Pork tenderloin, trimmed of fat	34
Beef, sirloin	34
Tuna, packed in water	28
Fish (cod, flounder, haddock)	21–30
Eggs, 2 large	14
Cottage cheese, low-fat, 1/2 cup	14
Milk, fat-free, 1 cup	8

essential amino acids; therefore, they are often called "complete" protein foods. These foods provide adequate protein to meet the body's protein needs, and it is relatively easy for both men and women to meet their daily protein requirements by eating them in fairly small amounts.

Let's look at an example of how a 130-pound woman can meet her protein requirement of 47 grams per day by eating animal sources of protein. Using Table 1, we can figure out what combinations of foods she can eat to meet that requirement. For example, if she eats

4 ounces tuna = 28 grams,
1/2 cup cottage cheese = 14 grams,
and 1 cup fat-free milk = 8 grams,

she will get a total of 50 grams of protein. As you can see, this woman's daily protein needs can easily be met by eating just these three sources of animal protein. It is no more challenging for men to meet their protein needs, even though they need more than women, since men tend to eat more than women, anyway.

The main problem with animal protein is that you get more than you bargain for. Animal sources of protein are often high in fat, primarily saturated fat. Saturated fat, in turn, is responsible for raising blood cholesterol levels, which can lead to heart disease. Because the majority of our protein intake comes from animal sources, it's really no surprise that our fat intake has increased, as well. In fact, some animal foods such as cheese and processed meats contain more calories from fat than from protein. It's important, therefore, to make sure you choose the leanest forms of animal protein foods to avoid the dangers of excess fat in your diet, which include obesity, heart disease, and cancer.

Protein from Plants?

Believe it or not, plants also contain protein, in addition to carbohydrate. In fact, someone who is a vegetarian probably gets his or her protein from plant foods. You may be curious (or even somewhat skeptical) about these plant proteins—just where *are* they found? A primary source of plant protein is *legumes*, or dried beans and peas. Examples are kidney beans, chickpeas (garbanzo beans), black beans, soybeans, lentils, and split peas. One-half cup of dried beans or peas contains 8 grams of protein, which is the amount of protein found in 1 ounce of meat, poultry, or fish.

Other sources of plant proteins are soy foods (tofu, soy milk, soy cheese, etc.), nuts, seeds, and "meat analogs," which are vegetarian-style versions of typical meat foods, such as burgers, hot dogs, and sausage. Meat analogs may be made from soybeans, vegetables, and/or grain foods, such as oatmeal. Remember that these foods eaten by themselves will not supply you with all of those essential amino acids we mentioned earlier. But you can get the essential amino acids by combining them with other foods. Turning up your nose at this point? Well, some very common things that you probably already eat contain combinations that make complete proteins; for example:

- peanut butter and jelly sandwiches
- black beans and rice
- vegetarian chili

- refried beans and tortilla chips
- minestrone soup
- hummus (chickpea spread) and pita bread

The beans or nuts and the grain foods—bread, rice, pasta, or tortillas—complement each other. When they are paired up, they provide you with protein just like that found in meats. And you don't need to combine them at the same meal. You can meet your protein requirements by eating a variety of foods over the course of the day.

Why would you want to eat plant protein foods instead of animal protein foods? Well, for several reasons. First, plant-based meals tend to be healthier for you. You already know that many animal protein foods are high in both total fat and saturated fat; plant protein foods are lower in fat, low in saturated fat, and contain more fiber. Second, plant-based meals add variety to your weekly menus. And third, meatless meals can be easy on your budget; plant protein foods are much less expensive than meat, poultry, or fish.

The Upside and Downside of Protein

The Role of Protein in Diabetic Kidney Disease

Kidney disease, called *nephropathy,* is one complication of diabetes. The kidneys act like filters in the body, working to remove toxic substances from the blood while retaining beneficial substances. The substances that are removed are excreted in the urine. Diabetes, particularly diabetes that is not well controlled, can damage the small filtering units of the kidney called *glomeruli*. Normally, glomeruli act to retain particles, such as protein, from being expelled in the urine. If these are damaged, as in the case of diabetes, protein molecules can slip through and enter the urine.

We know how important protein is for staying healthy. But for people with kidney disease, sometimes eating large amounts of protein is too much of a good thing; in fact, a high-protein diet can be downright harmful. Although there are still some conflicting opinions about the role of protein in kidney disease, there are good studies showing that a lower-protein diet may actually prevent kidney disease from worsening. People with end-stage renal failure (advanced kidney disease) often feel much better when they follow a lower-protein diet, since fewer nitrogenous wastes (wastes created when the body processes protein) build up in their blood. (Too much nitrogenous waste can be the result of a high protein intake and can make you feel nauseated and fatigued.)

Many physicians and dietitians recommend that people with diabetes who have early nephropathy start to cut back on their protein intake. Does this mean you should stop eating protein? Of course not. A low-protein diet must be carefully planned, preferably by a registered dietitian, to make sure you don't eat too little protein. A lower-protein diet does mean, however, that you need to eat smaller portions of meat, poultry, and fish, as well as limit the amount of dairy foods, such as milk, cheese, yogurt, and eggs, that you eat. There is some evidence that eating vegetable protein foods may be less harmful to the kidneys than eating animal protein foods. If you are following a lower-protein diet already and would like to try more plant-based meals, speak with your dietitian.

Too *Little* Protein?

So far, you've learned that people tend to eat too much protein and that too much protein may not be so healthy, especially for people with diabetes and kidney problems. What about not eating enough protein? Is this possible in a country known for thick steaks, fried chicken, and clambakes? Unfortunately, protein malnutrition is common in some Third World countries that are unable to feed their citizens adequately. However, the U.S. also has groups of people at risk for protein malnutrition, including low-income families, pregnant women who do not eat enough, alcoholics, and—at highest risk—older adults. Data from the National Health and Nutrition Examination Survey indicate that up to 25% of older Americans do not consume the RDA for protein; in fact, these people may be eating only half of the protein they need.

An elderly person who lives on a diet of "tea and toast" may lose lean body mass, which is mostly muscle. This, in turn, can lead to loss of strength and decreased muscle contraction. Insufficient protein intake can also impair the immune system, making that person more susceptible to disease and lengthening the recovery time from an illness or surgery. Obviously, older people need to make sure they eat a variety of foods, including poultry, fish, lean meats, dairy products, and/or legumes to ensure they consume enough of this important nutrient.

Weight Loss and High-Protein Diets

High-protein, low-carbohydrate diets have been around for several decades. Remember Dr. Atkins' Diet Revolution? The Stillman Diet? The Scarsdale Diet? The Beverly Hills Diet? The arrival of the nineties brought a fresh batch of "new" diet books—*The Zone, Protein Power, Healthy for Life, and Dr. Atkins' New Diet Revolution*—many of which tout the same claims as their older cousins. The underlying premise for most of these books is that a low-fat, high-carbohydrate diet can actually make you fat, because carbohydrate causes a release of insulin, which, in turn, leads to fat storage. What many readers who are desperate for the quick, easy solution to permanent weight loss do not realize is that there are no good studies showing that insulin causes weight gain. Unfortunately, they may be lead to believe that these lower-carbohydrate, higher-protein diets are the answer to their weight-loss woes, particularly when they actually do lose weight.

How can we explain the weight loss that does result from these diets? Well, what they have in common is that they all manage to cut calories, some more drastically than others. There really is no special magic: Anytime you decrease your caloric intake, weight loss will result. Keep in mind, too, that some of these diets have much more fat, especially saturated fat, than we should be consuming, which may spell trouble for your arteries down the road. Plus, if you follow the advice of some of these books, you'll find yourself following strict rules as to what times you can eat, what you can eat, and what combinations of foods you can eat together. Once again, there is no solid evidence backing up these claims.

Remember that, right now, there is no quick, super-easy way to shed those pounds. Eating right and exercising are still key. What you choose to eat makes a big difference. All leading health authorities still maintain that we need between 50–60% of our calories from carbohydrates, 15–20% from protein, and 30% or less from fat. So far, this seems to be the magic formula, especially when you eat whole-grain foods, fruits and vegetables, and lean protein sources. Oh, and don't forget to take that 30-minute walk!

Here's What You Can Do

1. **Calculate your own daily protein requirements.** As stated above, the RDA is 0.8 grams of protein for every kilogram of body weight. If working with kilograms is confusing for you, use the chart below to figure out how much protein *you* need every day. Keep in mind, too, that protein requirements are based on a healthy body weight, not necessarily how much you actually weigh. In other words, this doesn't mean that you need more protein if you are overweight. Multiply your (healthy) body weight in pounds by the appropriate number below to determine your daily protein requirements:

Adults 19 years and over	0.36
Pregnant women	0.62
Lactating women	0.53

your weight _____ × number from above _____
= _____ grams

2. **Keep your portion sizes in check.** Men and women need no more than about 3 to 6 ounces of protein each day. Three ounces is about the size of a deck of playing cards. So if your idea of a decent size piece of steak is 12 ounces—which is more like four decks of cards—you might want to cut back a little.

3. **Choose lean sources of protein.** Ideally, lower-fat protein foods have no more than 3 grams of total fat per serving. Try lower-fat versions of cheeses and processed meats. And incorporate plant-protein foods into your meal plan.

4. **Eat at least one meatless meal per week.** How about trying vegetable lasgagne, beans and rice, or soy burgers? Serve pasta as the main dish instead of as a side to chicken or veal. Toss some tofu into your stir-fry or just leave out the meat. Meatless meals don't have to be bland or boring!

5. **Talk to a dietitian.** A registered dietitian can help you learn how to combine plant-based foods to make sure you eat complete proteins, learn how to eat enough protein without eating too much fat, and how to balance your meal plan so that you are not eating more protein than your body needs.

6. **Don't fall for fad diets.** Talk to your health care provider before you buy into a high-protein, low-carbohydrate diet. If you want to lose weight, your health care provider and dietitian can help you adjust your meal plan to lose weight safely.

Summary

In this chapter, you've learned that protein is an essential nutrient—without it, we wouldn't survive. Protein is found in an abundant supply in foods such as poultry, seafood, meats, dairy foods, and even plant foods such as dried beans and peas. Most people in the U.S., with a few exceptions, eat enough protein. Too much protein, however, is not healthy, especially for people with diabetes and nephropathy. Once again, by eating a variety of foods and aiming for the RDA of protein, you can rest assured that you will get enough.

Your Turn

Now it's your turn to recall some key points from this chapter. Let's see how you do!

1. People with kidney disease should not eat any protein. True or false?
2. List three different animal protein foods:

   (1) _____

   (2) _____

   (3) _____
3. List three different plant protein foods:

   (1) _____

   (2) _____

   (3) _____
4. Plan to eat one meatless meal during the upcoming week.

   (Name of the meal you plan to try: _____
   _____)

See APPENDIX A for the answers.

5

Fat

Dennis: I can't believe I'm here. Aside from having diabetes, I have always been perfectly healthy. I received a call from my doctor after my last checkup telling me that my 'bad' cholesterol was too high and my 'good' cholesterol was too low. I don't even know what these words mean or how to change my way of eating. I know eggs and red meat have cholesterol in them, so if I avoid these, will my levels come down?

Dietitian: It isn't just avoiding specific foods, it's your overall fat intake over a period of time that makes a difference. When your cholesterol levels are too high, we teach you how to decrease your intake of fat, not just cholesterol. People with

M Y T H :

People with diabetes do not have to worry about eating fat because it doesn't have much of an effect on blood glucose.

diabetes are at a higher risk of developing hardening or blockage of the arteries, heart disease, and stroke than people without diabetes. Therefore, it is important that you know how the types and amounts of fat you eat play a role in increasing these health risks.

Dennis: I've also gained some weight in the last few years and have been so busy at work that I am forced to eat many meals on the run. My activity level has also suffered. So I guess we have to add weight loss to the list as well.

Dietitian: The good news is that when you cut down on your fat intake, you will also get rid of a lot of calories in the process. Fat contains more than twice as many calories as carbohydrate and protein. The good news is that you don't have to think of eating 'low fat' as something you have to do in addition to eating healthy. The same guidelines that help you eat healthfully will help you reduce your fat intake as well.

Dennis: Well, I guess it's about time I started concentrating on my health and taking the time to plan what and when I'm going to eat every day. I guess no more fast food.

Dietitian: Giving up all your favorite foods is not the goal. Everyone needs *some* fat for good health. Let's discuss how you can still fit in your favorite high-fat foods but limit how often you eat them.

What's Next?

Once Dennis learned how to determine whether a food was high in fat and how to read food labels, he found that he didn't have to give up his favorite high-fat foods completely. If he limited how often and how much of these foods he ate, they could still be part of his overall healthy food intake. Dennis also learned that some types of fat are healthier than others, although all fats are high in calories—even the "good" fats. By decreasing his fat intake, especially his saturated fat intake, Dennis was able to lower his "bad" cholesterol and increase his "good" cholesterol. He also lost 7 pounds in 1 month.

The Old and the New

In the days before insulin, people with diabetes were told to get about 70% of their daily calories from fat. Because fat was high in calories and was known to have the least effect on blood glucose, it was the one nutrient that they could eat to ensure enough calories and still attempt to control their blood glucose. Common sources of fat in the so-called diabetic diet included lots of cream, butter, oil, lard, mayonnaise, whole milk, nuts, and bacon along with eggs, cheese, and peanut butter.

The discovery of insulin, however, allowed people with diabetes to increase their intake of carbohydrate, thereby lowering their intake of fat. In 1950, the nutrition recommendation for fat intake was 40% of total daily calories. That was less than in the pre-insulin days, and it was the start of a downward trend. By 1971, recommendations for fat dropped to 35% of calories. And by 1986, people with diabetes were told to consume less than 30% of their daily calories from fat. This decrease was fueled by research studies that related fat to the number-one cause of death in our country: heart disease.

Research had also shown that lowering blood cholesterol levels could lower your chance of having problems with the heart and blood vessels.

Since 1994, the American Diabetes Association's nutrition recommendations have stated that there is no one standard "diet" for people with diabetes. The distribution of calories from fat and carbohydrate should be tailored to the individual. The percentage of calories from fat will depend on the individual's goals for blood fat levels, as well as for weight. People with normal blood fat levels who are at a healthy weight may want to get 30% or less of their total daily calories from fat. Those with abnormal blood fat levels or who are overweight may want to get only 20–25% of their total daily calories from fat.

What Is Fat?

Have you ever heard the term "blood lipids"? Lipid is simply a word used for fat. Most of the fats in our food or our body are called *triglycerides*. Another member of the lipid family is *cholesterol*. When we talk about reducing cardiovascular disease or high cholesterol levels, we talk about cutting down on *dietary fat* (which includes triglycerides, saturated or unsaturated) and *dietary cholesterol*. When we talk about the blood test done at the doctor's office called a lipid profile, we are talking about *blood fat* (or triglycerides) and *blood cholesterol*. Basically, we are talking about fats in food and fats in the blood, and more specifically, how to change and decrease the fats in the food so we have less fat in the blood. So when your doctor tells you that you have hyperlipidemia (a high lipid level), it actually means that you have too much cholesterol or fat in your blood.

We often hear of fats categorized as "good" and "bad." What this is really referring to is the two different forms of fats: saturated and unsaturated. Fats are distinguished by their level of saturation or "fullness." This all has to do with the chemical structure of a fat and how solid its structure is. Saturated fats and trans fats are more solid at room temperature than unsaturated fats. Research has shown that foods high in saturated fat cause blood cholesterol levels to rise more than foods containing cholesterol that are not also high in fat.

What Is Cholesterol?

Cholesterol is a fat-like, waxy substance that is found in specific foods we eat. Probably the most important fact about cholesterol is that it is *only* found in animal foods. These animal foods include meat, fish, poultry, eggs, and dairy products. Plant foods do not contain cholesterol. Because the body produces cholesterol, it is not *essential* in our diet. So, we get cholesterol in two ways: by eating animal foods and by producing it in our bodies, primarily by the *liver*. Blood cholesterol comes mostly from fats in foods, saturated fats in particular.

Fat and cholesterol are traveling companions in the bloodstream. They are transported through the blood by a protein-carrier called a *lipoprotein*. Generally, you can think of a lipoprotein as a wagon carrying fat and cholesterol. Because blood is a water-based substance and fat is an oil-based substance, fat cannot mix with water or travel in the bloodstream without help. This means that fat and cholesterol are carried inside of a protein particle (the wagon) through the bloodstream.

There are two major lipoproteins that your doctor measures and has probably mentioned: high-density lipoprotein (HDL) and low-density lipoprotein (LDL). The more protein in the lipoprotein, the less fat it can carry, or the higher the density. Because it carries more protein and less fat and cholesterol, HDL can carry the cholesterol and fat away from the arteries and cells and back to the liver for recycling or elimination. Therefore, HDL is sometimes called the "good" or "healthy" cholesterol. The more fat in the lipoprotein, the less protein, or the lower the density. Because it carries less protein and more fat and cholesterol, LDL can deposit cholesterol and fat in the arteries and cells, causing a buildup in the body. Therefore, LDL is sometimes referred to as the "bad" or "less healthy" cholesterol.

LDL is closely related to heart disease. If your LDL cholesterol level is high, you are at a higher risk for heart attack. HDL seems to have a protective effect on the heart, however. If your HDL cholesterol level is high, you are at less risk for heart disease.

Where Is Fat Found?

We mentioned previously that fats are categorized according to their structure and level of saturation, or fullness. We also noted that the saturated or solid fats in the diet are the fats that cause blood cholesterol levels to rise. Let's now see which fats are the most "heart healthy" and which are the most "heart harmful."

The most important thing to know about healthy fats and harmful fats is that they both contain the same amount of calories. So it is essential that you be aware of the quantity as well as the quality of the fat you eat if you want to lower your weight *and* cholesterol levels. Next, we will look at the different types of fat and where these fats are found. But keep in mind that no fat or oil is made up of just one kind of fat. For example, although olive oil is mostly monounsaturated fat, about 20% of it is saturated fat. The fats are listed in descending order from more healthy to more harmful, according to current research.

- **Monounsaturated fats** are liquid at room temperature and are found in olive, canola, and peanut oils; avocados; nuts; and olives. These help to *lower* LDL cholesterol and possibly *raise* HDL cholesterol levels. Most of your fat intake should come from monounsaturated fats.
- **Polyunsaturated fats** are liquid at room temperature and are found in corn, safflower, sesame, and soybean oils. These lower both your LDL and HDL levels (remember, the goal is to raise HDL, not lower it).
- **Omega-3** is a type of polyunsaturated fat found in fatty fish such as mackerel, salmon, tuna, sardines, and bluefish. Flaxseed oil is also a good source. It is *not* recommended that you take fish oil supplements, but rather that you eat fish at meals at least two or three times per week. Omega-3 fatty acids help to prevent clotting and stickiness on artery walls.
- **Saturated fats** are solid at room temperature. These fats come mainly from animal products and are found in butter, meat, lard, poultry skin, whole milk, cheese,

sour cream, cream cheese, and yogurt. They are also found in coconut, cocoa butter (chocolate), palm oils, and palm kernel oil. They lower HDL and raise LDL.

■ **Trans fats** are partially solid at room temperature. These come from the polyunsaturated vegetable oils listed above. Through a process called hydrogenation, liquid oil goes through a chemical process in which it is changed from a liquid into a solid or partially solid fat. These fats are found in products such as margarine and shortening, cakes, cookies, crackers, donuts, chips, and other baked goods. Trans fats are common because they give foods a longer shelf life. They raise your blood cholesterol levels like saturated fats. They lower HDL and raise LDL.

Because both saturated fats and trans fats can raise your cholesterol level, they should be carefully monitored and used in moderation. Keep this in mind as a general guideline: the softer or more liquid the fat, the better.

Why Do We Need Fat?

Fat does have usefulness and is necessary for good health. Fat is our storage form of calories, or energy, and is accessible from storage (mostly in the fat cells) if food is not available or if extra energy is needed for activity. Because fats have more than twice as many calories as carbohydrate and protein, fats can store more than twice as many calories in a small space. Although carbohydrate can be stored in smaller amounts, a person with diabetes does not have the ability to store carbohydrate and then quickly make it available for extra calories in the amount or at the exact time it might be needed. For survival purposes, fat storage is beneficial as a concentrated source of energy, but too much storage in the absence of physical activity or work can be harmful when it leads to overweight or obesity.

A layer of fat under the skin works as an insulator for any variables in temperatures we might encounter, and it works as a cushion for all the important organs in our bodies. Fat also helps to make up the outer structure of all of our body cells and forms a protective barrier. If your hands are in constant contact with strong soap and water, for example, you can damage the protective fat layer in the skin cells, which eventually leaves the skin dry and cracked.

One of the most important functions of fat is providing important nutrients, namely, the fat-soluble vitamins A, D, E, and K. These fat-soluble vitamins can mainly be found in foods that contain fat and can only be carried through the blood to cells in the body by fat. Fat also provides flavor, tenderness, aroma, and palatability.

Cholesterol is made by our liver and also has some essential functions. It is used in the digestion of fats and as a part of certain hormones. It helps form vitamin D, and it makes up the outer structure of all body cells.

The Upside and Downside of Fat

Fat has received particularly bad reviews in recent years. Although many Americans need to cut down their fat intake, some have become fat-phobic. They are eating less than 20% of their total daily calories from fat, and to make up for the calories lost from fat, they end up eating too many calories, mostly from carbohydrate. So as our fat intake has decreased in the U.S., from 40% of our total daily calories to less than 33%, the total number of calories consumed per person has risen 7%. Health experts are now thinking that if you eat too little fat, maybe a little more should be added as long as it's coming from unsaturated fats, preferably monounsaturated.

The Downside

1. **Extra calories.** Because fat has more than twice as many calories as carbohydrate and protein, even small amounts can add up to pounds. There are 9 calories in every gram of fat, compared to 4 calories in each gram of carbohydrate or protein.
2. **Clogged arteries.** If you eat too much saturated fat, you may end up clogging your arteries and eventually cutting off the supply of blood to the heart.
3. **Chronic disease link.** A high-fat diet increases the risk not only of heart disease and obesity, but also of high blood pressure and possibly some types of cancer.
4. **Small serving sizes.** Serving sizes for most fat require that you eat very small portions. For example, 1 level teaspoon of margarine, butter, all types of oils, and mayonnaise equals 1 serving size. A serving size of regular salad dressing is 1 level tablespoon. Light or fat-free versions of these foods are better choices if you are unable to stick to the small serving sizes—as long as you check out the carbohydrate content in these products.
5. **Fat-free not calorie-free.** In low-fat and fat-free products, fat is usually replaced with carbohydrate. Therefore, the total number of calories often is not reduced, and if eaten in large amounts, these products can raise blood glucose.

The Upside

1. **Food additive.** Fat provides flavor and enhances taste. It adds moistness, acts as a tenderizer and preservative, and contributes to the creamy, crunchy, or crispy mouth-feel of foods. It is also responsible for wonderfully potent aromas.
2. **Unlimited storage capacity.** Stored fat provides energy needed during exercise or long periods of food deprivation.
3. **Protection for the body.** Fat keeps the body warm and cushions it against shock and injury.
4. **Carrier of important vitamins.** Fat carries important vitamins, namely vitamins A, D, E, and K.

Here's What You Can Do

1. **Ask your doctor for a lipid profile on a yearly basis or more often if you have hyperlipidemia.** A lipid profile is a blood test done in a laboratory that requires a small sample of your blood. This profile will tell you what your blood levels are for total cholesterol, LDL cholesterol, HDL cholesterol, and triglycerides. Compare your results with the following desired levels:

   - Total cholesterol: less than 200 mg/dl
   - HDL cholesterol: more than 45 mg/dl
   - LDL cholesterol: less than 100 mg/dl
   - Triglycerides: less than 200 mg/dl

2. **Make an appointment with a registered dietitian to determine how much fat you should be taking in each day.** This is different for all people. It depends on many factors such as weight, age, activity level, cul-

tural background, total daily calorie intake, laboratory values, and family history.

3. **Investigate your risk factors for heart disease.** The following is a list of the major risk factors for heart disease. Those risk factors that are either controllable or have a relationship with food intake are indicated with an asterisk (*).

- Men, over 45 years old; women, over 55 years old or premature menopause without estrogen replacement therapy
- Family history of premature heart disease
- Cigarette smoking*
- High blood pressure: over 140/90 mmHg or taking hypertension medication*
- Low HDL: less than 35 mg/dl*
- High LDL: 130 mg/dl or more*
- Low physical activity level*
- Obesity*
- Diabetes*

4. **Remember moderation.** No foods have to be cut out completely. Some may just have to be eaten less often and in smaller amounts.

5. **Substitute unsaturated fats for many saturated fats.** Use more low-fat or light versions of salad dressings, mayonnaise, cream cheese, sour cream, and milk.

6. **Instead of frying, broil, steam, bake, or grill foods.**

7. **Remove skin from poultry (either before or after cooking) and trim the fat off of meat.**

8. **Use only half the amount of oil called for in recipes.** If you do use oil, use a monounsaturated oil such as olive, canola, or peanut oil, or purchase these in non-stick sprays.

9. **Read labels.** The upper part of the food label will tell you how many of the calories are coming from fat. As long as your intake of fat in a day is only 20–30% of your total calories, it is okay if an individual food is higher. Total fat grams per serving and how much of the total fat is coming from saturated fat are listed just below the calories. Some manufacturers might even tell you the amount of mono- and polyunsaturated fats. You will not see trans fats listed on the label, but you should be able to find evidence of them if you look at the ingredient list and see the words *hydrogenated* or *partially hydrogenated* vegetable oil. Also, look at the nutrient claims for fat and remember the fat claims listed on the label only apply to *one* serving.

Summary

It's important for all of us to take control of our health by decreasing our risk of heart disease. Lowering your health risks requires regular visits with your diabetes team members. Your team will help you to be well informed about healthy eating. Make a list of your risk factors for heart disease, and work on those factors that you do have some control over, such as cigarette smoking and activity level. Also, focus on those risk factors that are controllable *and* have a relationship with food, such as obesity, high blood pressure, diabetes, low HDL, and high LDL.

Your best bet is to be realistic and flexible. Make small changes over time and balance your food choices over the period of a day. Remember, the amount of food you eat has more of an effect than the type of food you eat.

Your Turn

Now it's your turn to recall some key points from this chapter. Let's see how you do!

1. Most of the fats in our food and our body are called
   _____.
2. A _____ fat is more solid at room temperature than an unsaturated fat, which is liquid at room temperature.
3. High-density lipoprotein (HDL) is considered more healthy because it carries more protein and less _____. Low-density lipoprotein (LDL) is considered less healthy because it carries less _____ and more fat.
4. Which of the following statements refer to *positive* roles fat plays?

   ___protects our major organs

   ___helps lower cholesterol levels

   ___prevents dry skin

   ___maintains our body temperature

   ___provides lots of calories

   ___stores vitamins A, D, E, and K

   ___intensifies the taste of foods

   ___provides fiber

See APPENDIX A for the answers.

6

Sugar Substitutes

Erin: I have always wondered why sometimes my blood glucose is elevated after I eat some sugar-free foods, and often my stomach aches. What does this all mean?

Dietitian: You might be surprised to learn that sugar-free does not necessarily mean calorie-free or carbohydrate-free, and that some sugar substitutes may not have a significant benefit over regular sugars, such as table sugar.

Erin: Do you mean that I can't eat unlimited amounts of sugar-free foods?

Dietitian: Although some sugar substitutes don't have any calories, other sugar substitutes do provide calories and carbohydrate. These can affect your blood

MYTH:

People with diabetes should only eat foods sweetened with sugar substitutes instead of sugar.

glucose and even your weight. What this means is that most foods with sugar substitutes must be counted into your carbohydrate allowance in your meal plan. Furthermore, when eaten in large quantities, some of these sugar substitutes may have a laxative effect.

Erin: Well, if I still have to count some of these sugar substitutes as part of my carbohydrate allowance, couldn't I use my carbohydrate allowance on *any* food?

Dietitian: Absolutely! The choice is yours. Because we know that a carbohydrate is a carbohydrate, you can spend your carbohydrate grams or exchanges on whatever foods you choose.

What's Next?

Erin was surprised to learn that whereas *nonnutritive* (no-calorie) sweeteners (aspartame, saccharin, acesulfame potassium, and sucralose) do allow people with diabetes to enjoy the sweet taste that most humans desire in foods without affecting blood glucose or weight, the *nutritive* (calorie-containing) sweeteners (sugar alcohols, fructose, polydextrose, and maltodextrin) do provide both calories and carbohydrate. Erin was taught that although some nutritive sugar substitutes, such as sugar alcohols, may produce a slightly lower rise in blood glucose, this is because they are poorly absorbed from the digestive tract. However, they must still be counted as part of the carbohydrate allowance in her meal plan. She also learned that nutrition recommendations by the American Diabetes Association state that foods made with nutritive sugar substitutes may not have a significant advantage over foods sweetened with regular sugars either in cutting down calories and carbohydrate or improving blood glucose.

The Old and the New

So-called diabetic foods began emerging over 100 years ago because of the numerous and often unattainable food restrictions of the "diabetic diet." Because people with diabetes enjoyed sweet foods just as much as those without diabetes, sugar substitutes became a necessity. Over the past 40 years, sugar substitutes have become common ingredients because of the thinking that sugar should be avoided because of its perceived rapid absorption and resulting rise in blood glucose. They are added to a wide variety of foods enjoyed by most people with diabetes. In addition, many of these foods are also being used by those without diabetes, mainly for weight control.

Today, with our current knowledge of sugar and its effects on blood glucose, we know that sugar substitutes and regular sugars, such as sucrose and fructose, are all acceptable sources of sweetness. However, because not all sugar substitutes are calorie free, they are not necessarily beneficial for weight loss or blood glucose control. Many people with diabetes assume that all foods containing sugar substitutes can be eaten as "free foods," and this may lead to problems with blood glucose and weight control. As with any food that contributes calories and carbohydrate, nutritive sweeteners still have to be accounted for in the meal plan.

Before 1970, our goals for food were mostly focused on safety and on nutritional deficiencies. Today, our goals for food have changed. They now focus on how food relates to health promotion and disease prevention. Because of our plentiful food supply and the resulting overweight and obesity issues in our country, the perceived need for low-calorie foods is high. Let's take a look at the facts so that if you do choose to use sugar substitutes, you will know their potential effects on your blood glucose and weight.

Here Are the Facts

Sweeteners fall into two categories: nutritive and nonnutritive. These terms differentiate those sweeteners with and without calories. Other terms used to describe sweeteners are *sugar substitutes, sugar replacers,* and *alternative sweeteners.*

Nonnutritive: High-Intensity Sweeteners

Currently, four high-intensity sweeteners are regulated for food use: *saccharin, aspartame, acesulfame K,* and *sucralose.* All are identified as food additives, and saccharin is the most widely used. It takes very little of these sweeteners to obtain maximum sweetening ability. These high-intensity sweeteners offer the benefit of sweet taste without calories, carbohydrate, or response from blood glucose, and they don't promote tooth decay. The current trend is to blend different high-intensity sweeteners so that less sweetener is needed to obtain a sweeter, improved taste. For example, a blend might include aspartame and acesulfame K and still not provide calories.

Because high-intensity sweeteners are food additives, manufacturers must provide information about a sweetener's safety limit, which is known as the acceptable daily intake (ADI). The ADI is the estimated amount of sweetener, based on body weight, that a person can safely consume every day over a lifetime.

Saccharin

Saccharin has no calories and is 200 to 700 times sweeter than table sugar (sucrose). It is heat-stable and may be used in cooking. It is not broken down by the body and is eliminated unchanged. Saccharin is used as a tabletop sweetener (Sweet'n Low) as well as in chewing gum, cosmetics, medications, foods, and beverages. The ADI is 5 milligrams per kilogram of body weight. One packet of the tabletop version contains 40 milligrams.

Aspartame

Better known as NutraSweet, aspartame has 4 calories per gram, but it can be used in such small amounts that the amount of calories it adds to a product is negligible. It is 160 to 220 times sweeter than table sugar. Aspartame is not heat-stable and may lose its sweetness after long exposure to high temperatures. It is rapidly broken down in the digestive tract and does not build up in the body at recommended intakes. It is used as a tabletop sweetener (Equal and other brand names) as well as in carbonated beverages, powdered drinks, yogurt, gelatin, cereals, and frozen desserts. The ADI is 50 milligrams per kilogram of body weight. One packet of the tabletop version contains 37 milligrams.

Acesulfame K

Produced under the brand name Sunette, acesulfame K (or acesulfame potassium) has no calories. It is 200 times sweeter than table sugar. Acesulfame K is heat-stable and may be used in cooking. It is not broken down by the body and is eliminated unchanged. It is used as a tabletop sweetener (Sweet One, Swiss Sweet) and as an additive in chewing gum, confections, desserts, yogurt, sauces, and alcoholic beverages. The ADI of acesulfame K is 15 milligrams per kilogram of body weight. A packet of the tabletop version contains 50 milligrams.

Sucralose

Marketed under the brand name Splenda, sucralose has no calories and is 600 times sweeter than table sugar. It is heat-stable and may be used in cooking. It is not broken down by the body and is eliminated unchanged. It is used as a tabletop sweetener as well as in desserts, confections, and nonalcoholic drinks. The ADI is 5–15 milligrams per kilogram of body weight. A packet of the tabletop version contains 5 milligrams.

Nutritive Sweeteners: Sugar Alcohols

Nutritive sweeteners include sugar, fructose, corn syrup, and many others, as described in chapter 2. Sugar substitutes such as sugar alcohols, maltodextrin, and polydextrose are also nutritive sweeteners. Although the Food and Drug Administration (FDA) defines high-intensity nonnutritive sweeteners as food additives, it considers nutritive sweeteners such as sugar alcohols to be "Generally Recognized as Safe" (GRAS) ingredients.

The sugar alcohols most commonly found in foods are *sorbitol, mannitol, xylitol, isomalt,* and *hydrogenated starch hydrolysates (HSH)*. Sugar alcohols come from plant products such as fruits and berries. The carbohydrate in the plant products is altered through a chemical process that results in the formation of sugar alcohols. These sugar substitutes provide somewhat fewer calories and less carbohydrate than sugar sweeteners, producing a smaller rise in blood glucose and decreasing the risk of tooth decay. The sugar alcohols are also absorbed more slowly and incompletely from the digestive tract, often producing a laxative effect if eaten excessively.

Unfortunately, people with diabetes often do eat excessive amounts of foods containing sugar alcohols, thinking they are "free foods" like those made with high-intensity sweeteners. When this happens, the sugar alcohols may contribute excessive calories and cause a rise in blood glucose. Therefore, even though sugar alcohols are considered reduced-calorie sweeteners, if their serving size is not observed and the calorie and carbohydrate contents are not accounted for, they may provide no significant benefit over regular sugars, such as sucrose and fructose. Below you will find a description of the five nutritive sugar alcohols:

- **Sorbitol** is used in candies, chewing gum, jams and jellies, baked goods, and frozen confections. It provides 2.6 calories per gram and is 50–70% as sweet as table sugar.
- **Mannitol** is used as a dusting agent for chewing gum and as a bulking agent in powdered foods. It provides 1.6 calories per gram and is 50–70% as sweet as table sugar.

- **Xylitol** is used in chewing gum, candies, pharmaceuticals, and hygiene products. It provides 2.4 calories per gram and is as sweet as sugar.
- **Isomalt** is used in confections and/or as a bulking agent. It provides 2 calories per gram and is 45–65% as sweet as table sugar.
- **Hydrogenated starch hydrolysates** (HSH or maltitol syrup) are used in confections and/or as bulking agents. They provide 3 calories per gram and are 24–50% as sweet as table sugar.

Blending

Sugar substitutes, both nutritive and nonnutritive, are often blended together. Sugar alcohols are usually less sweet than table sugar but do add bulk to products, as do regular sugars. High-intensity sweeteners provide a concentrated sweetness in a very small volume but no bulk. So a blend might include a mixture of several sugar alcohols as well as a high-intensity sweetener. Therefore, if you see aspartame (nonnutritive) listed on the front of a package, you still have to look at the carbohydrate content to see if any sugar alcohols (nutritive) are blended with the aspartame. This blend does not constitute a free food and you will have to plan accordingly.

Here's What You Can Do

Because we now know that all sugar-free foods are not created equal, the first step when considering a sugar-free food is to check the food label. Below is a quick and easy way to find out if a high-intensity sweetener is the only sweetener in the product or if there is a blend of other sugars or sugar alcohols with the high-intensity sweetener. To avoid being misled, use the following guidelines:

1. Look immediately at the total carbohydrate in 1 serving size. If a serving has 5 grams or less of total carbohydrate, that food is counted as a free food. **You can stop right here.** However, free foods should still be limited to no more than 3–4 servings spread out over the day.
2. If the food has more than 5 grams of total carbohydrate, then the carbohydrate amount has to be counted as part of your carbohydrate allowance.
3. Because carbohydrate has the biggest impact on your blood glucose, you only need to focus on the amount of carbohydrate in a serving. However, if you focus on sugars (listed under total carbohydrate), you might be misled because you will likely see 0 grams. Because sugar alcohols do not have to be listed under sugars (they are sugar substitutes), looking only at sugar may lead you to believe that the food will not affect your blood glucose or weight. However, sugar alcohols or any other sugars *always* have to be included in the total carbohydrate grams. You will never be misled if you only focus on total carbohydrate grams.

Examples

Let's look at a couple of examples of sugar-free foods.

	Diet Soda (12-ounce can)	Sugar-Free Sandwich Cookies
Serving size	1 can	3 cookies
Total carbohydrate	0 grams	21 grams
Sugars	0 grams	0 grams
Sugar substitutes	Aspartame	Sorbitol, polydextrose, maltodextrin, aspartame

Which will affect your blood glucose, the soda or the cookies? If you look at total carbohydrate, you will see that although they are "sugar free," the cookies have enough carbohydrate to affect your blood glucose. The diet soda is a free food.

Commonly Asked Questions

Does "no sugar added" mean the same thing as "sugar free"? No. Both terms have different meanings. "Sugar free" means less than 0.5 grams of sugar per serving. This does not apply to sugar substitutes such as the sugar alcohols. "No sugar added" means that the processing and packing does not increase the sugar content over the amount naturally found in the ingredients. For example, an ice cream bar made with aspartame may be called "no sugar added" because it is sweetened with a sugar substitute instead of sucrose (table sugar). However, it cannot be called "sugar free" because the milk it's made with contains the natural sugar lactose.

Since it has calories and carbohydrate, can I use a sugar-free food sweetened with a sugar alcohol to treat low

blood glucose? No. It is not recommended that you use these foods as treatments for hypoglycemia (low blood glucose) because the carbohydrate in sugar alcohols is more slowly absorbed from the digestive tract and may not work quickly enough. Also, many of these foods have a lot of fat in a serving. Fat slows down stomach emptying and also does not work fast enough to raise your blood glucose.

I've always heard that if a food has 20 calories or less, it is considered a free food. Is this true? Yes, this is true. Earlier in the chapter, we stated that if a food has 5 grams or less of total carbohydrate, it is considered a free food. Each gram of carbohydrate provides 4 calories, so 5 grams of carbohydrate provides 20 calories. Therefore, both statements are correct.

Your Turn

Now it's your turn to recall some key points from this chapter. Let's see how you do!

1. Eating excess sugar-free foods can increase your blood glucose and weight. True or false?
2. A free food is any food with _____ grams of carbohydrate or less, or _____ calories or less, but should be limited to no more than _____ servings spread out over the day.
3. Sweeteners are defined in one of two categories: _____ or _____.
4. Which high-intensity sweetener is not heat stable and may become bitter to the taste after long exposure to

high temperatures? aspartame _____ saccharin _____
acesulfame K _____ sucralose _____

5. Go to the kitchen and look at some of the sugar-free foods (frozen desserts, candies, cookies, or beverages) you eat on a regular basis. Use the format below to see if you need to count these foods as part of your carbohydrate allowance:

Serving Size: _____

Total Carbohydrate: _____

Sugar: _____ (naturally occurring?)

Sugar Substitutes: _____

See APPENDIX A for the answers.

Carbohydrate Counting

David: I was recently married, and my wife, Louise, who is a nurse, is very supportive. She wanted to accompany me to my appointment today to update her knowledge about eating with diabetes. I have tried to use the exchange system numerous times during the 10 years that I have had diabetes, but it is too complicated and time-consuming. I am embarrassed to admit that I was never able to stick with this system, so I just gave up! How do other people with diabetes stick to it? I guess I'm just a bad diabetic.

Dietitian: Don't be so hard on yourself. No one is perfect. The main goal of living with diabetes is to maintain near-normal blood glucose levels by balancing your

MYTH:

People with diabetes must use the exchange system for meal planning to manage their diabetes.

food intake with your diabetes medications and activity levels. My goal as your dietitian is to help you and Louise make small changes in your eating that will improve your nutrition skills and blood glucose levels without totally altering your lifestyle.

David: But I've seen many dietitians over the years, and they seem so inflexible and judgmental. What is different now? And what is this 'carbohydrate counting' that Louise has been reading about?

Dietitian: Because nutrition is an essential—and often the most challenging—part of successful diabetes care, health professionals have come to realize that one diet *doesn't* fit all. You need a meal planning method that is appropriate for your personal lifestyle and cultural background. Carbohydrate counting, for example, is a method in which you keep track of how many carbohydrate foods you are eating at each meal and snack. Many people find this meal planning approach easier to follow because it allows them to fit in any food they like, as long as their overall eating is healthy.

David: Do you mean I don't have to give up all of my favorite family foods and be *hungry* all the time?

Dietitian: That's right. You, Louise, and I will work together to develop a meal planning option that you are able and willing to do—and most importantly, it will be one that is realistic for your lifestyle.

What's Next?

People like David who have had diabetes for many years will never forget the many restrictions placed on them and their food choices when they were first diagnosed. Often they were made to feel that they lacked willpower or were just plain cheating when they were unable to stick to a rigid diet given to them by their doctor.

Because of the many changes that have taken place in the diabetes and nutrition arena, we know today that there is no one "diabetic" or "ADA" diet. Research has provided health professionals with the opportunity to offer more flexible guidelines rather than rigid rules. Unfortunately, like David, many people with diabetes are unaware of these positive changes and new approaches. The dietitian was particularly happy that David's wife, Louise, accompanied him to the appointment, since she did most of the cooking and was his primary support person. As a nurse, Louise had learned about diabetes meal planning when she was in school, but she now wanted to learn the new nutrition guidelines that she had been reading about.

The first issue addressed by the dietitian was David's constant hunger. She explained that another important goal of nutrition therapy is to provide adequate calories either to maintain or attain a reasonable weight. Since David was a thin man in his thirties who worked at an active construction site, the dietitian wanted to assess his nutrition needs and ensure that he would receive enough calories. Next, the dietitian asked David about his favorite foods, his usual food intake, his workweek and weekend schedules, and his activity level so that she would be able to distribute his calories and carbohydrate in a realistic way. David was then made aware of the many meal planning options now available. They discussed which option would be the most realistic and compatible with his lifestyle.

After a couple of sessions with the dietitian to review the new guidelines and receive a solid education in how diabetes, food, and activity interact, David and Louise agreed that carbohydrate counting would be best suited for David to help him meet his nutrition goals. David's renewed interest in his diabetes self-management allowed him to learn how to interpret his blood glucose numbers and use this information when planning meals and snacks to gain better diabetes control.

The Old and the New

Until 1950, standard food lists specifying portion sizes for each individual food were not available. The doctor and the patient would have to spend hours calculating, measuring, eliminating, and guessing how much, when, and what to eat. Food choices were rigid and monotonous, eating outside of the home was impossible, and rarely could casseroles or mixed dishes be eaten. In 1950, The American Dietetic Association and the American Diabetes Association, together with the U.S. Public Health Service, devised a meal planning method using a food exchange system. This was simply a framework that grouped together foods that were similar in calories, carbohydrate, protein, and fat. This system allowed foods from the same group to be substituted for each other and was to be used universally so that everyone with diabetes would be using one uniform method to account for what they ate.

From this new method came preprinted tear-off sheets of standardized diets, which meant that health professionals did not have to spend time calculating individual meal plans. Unfortunately, these diet sheets did not take into account each individual's likes and dislikes, cultural background, or overall lifestyle. When a person with diabetes was unable to adhere to these diet sheets, she or he was thought to be noncompliant, unmotivated, or difficult.

The exchange system was updated and modified in 1976, 1986, and 1995, while still maintaining the basic framework developed in 1950. Each revision, although allowing for more food choices, still caused confusion for many patients and health professionals; some patients still were unable to follow their meal plans for any length of time.

The 1994 American Diabetes Association nutrition recommendations stated that choosing an appropriate meal planning method based on each person's ability, willingness, educational level, and nutritional needs was necessary. The exchange system could not be the only meal planning option available. When this system was developed in the 1950s, we did not have even half of the food choices that are available to us today. Furthermore, not only do we eat restaurant or take-out meals more often, but we incorporate many more convenience, frozen, and ethnic foods on a regular basis.

Here Are the Facts

Although other meal planning approaches have been around for many years, many people with diabetes still believe that the exchange system is the only method of meal planning. However, like David, many people with diabetes are curious to learn more about their options, and one option in particular: carbohydrate counting. This counting approach has evolved over the past several years to meet the demands of the person who wants to take charge of his or her diabetes self-management. Those people who are using diet and exercise alone or diabetes pills to control their diabetes can use this approach to help manage weight and blood glucose by regulating how much carbohydrate is eaten at each meal and snack. Those on insulin may also use this approach to coordinate food intake (mostly carbohydrate), exercise, and insulin, by matching the peak activity of the insulin with the peak levels of blood glucose.

The Diabetes Control and Complications Trial (DCCT), which began in the 1980s, was a large diabetes study that selected close to 1,500 people with type 1 diabetes to follow for a period of close to 10 years. The DCCT was able to demonstrate that *any* improvement in blood glucose control makes a difference in delaying the onset and progression of diabetes complications. Carbohydrate counting was one of four meal planning approaches used in the DCCT. Both patients and health professionals found that this system allowed more flexibility in food choices and helped with meeting diabetes self-management goals.

Simply stated, carbohydrate counting is a meal planning approach that focuses primarily on the total amount of carbohydrate. This is based on the premise that carbohydrate is converted to blood glucose (sugar) beginning about 15 minutes after the start of the meal, with the total carbohydrate from the meal being completely converted to blood glucose within the first 2 hours after the meal. The idea is that because 100% of carbohydrate is converted into blood glucose, eating an established amount of carbohydrate at each meal will keep your blood glucose level more consistent. As we learned in chapters 2 and 3, two forms of carbohydrate (starch and sugar) have about the same effect on blood glucose, so they can be substituted for each other.

Carbohydrate counting emphasizes the relationship between food, activity, blood glucose, and medication. It is less structured and less complex than the exchange diet because it focuses on only one nutrient. However, this does not mean that we can simply ignore protein and fat because they have less of an effect on blood glucose (58% and 10%, respectively). Healthy eating is still the main goal.

Exchange Lists Versus Carbohydrate Counting

Look at the chart below to see how exchanges can be converted to carbohydrate grams for carbohydrate counting.

Exchange System Approach	Carbohydrate Counting
1 starch	15 grams of carbohydrate
1 fruit	15 grams of carbohydrate
1 milk	15 grams of carbohydrate
1 vegetable	0 grams of carbohydrate
1 meat	0 grams of carbohydrate
1 fat	0 grams of carbohydrate

Note that although 1 vegetable exchange actually contains 5 grams of carbohydrate, much of that carbohydrate comes from fiber, which has little effect on blood glucose. Therefore, vegetables are not counted unless eaten in larger quantities. For example, 1/2 cup cooked carrots would not be counted as carbohydrate, but 1 1/2 cups cooked carrots would be counted as 15 grams of carbohydrate. Also, the amount of carbohydrate in 1 milk exchange is actually 12 grams, but it has been rounded up to 15 grams for carbohydrate counting purposes.

Budgeting Your Carbohydrate Allowance

Every person needs a certain amount of fuel from food each day. The bulk of this fuel comes from carbohydrate foods, although protein and fat contribute some. The carbohydrate foods make up our total daily carbohydrate *allowance*. Your daily carbohydrate allowance is the amount of carbohydrate you can *spend* during the day. It must be spread out, *budgeted*, between meals and snacks. The amount of carbohydrate in your budget for each meal or snack is more important than your allowance for the whole day.

Some foods (cereals, candy, desserts, and sodas, for example) contain more carbohydrate than other foods. Think of these foods as being more *expensive* because they require you to spend a large amount of your carbohydrate allowance when you choose them. For example, 1/4 cup of maple syrup has about 50 grams of carbohydrate, the same amount as more than three pancakes. The maple syrup might taste good, but the pancakes will fill you up and will supply more nutrients your body needs. How would you rather spend those 50 grams of carbohydrate? The main goal of carbohydrate counting is to budget your carbohydrate allowance wisely to get the most value from what you "buy."

Here's What You Can Do

We now know that the types of foods that you eat and the amounts of foods that you eat, especially carbohydrate foods, determine how high and how fast your blood glucose level goes up. It is important to know how many grams of carbohydrate you will be eating at each meal and snack. This will help you know what to expect from your blood glucose. Many people think the carbohydrate counting approach is more precise than the exchange system for meal planning.

Here are some tips to help you get on the fast road to carbohydrate counting:

1. Set up a visit with a registered dietitian (RD) who is also a certified diabetes educator (CDE). This health professional will work with you to determine how much food your body needs each day based on your age, height, weight, and activity level, while taking into consideration your favorite foods, your cultural background, and your lifestyle. There is no set amount of carbohydrate that is recommended for all people with diabetes.

2. The dietitian will help you determine your carbohydrate allowance—the total number of carbohydrate grams you can spend at each meal and snack—and will help you learn how to budget your allowance.

3. Practice learning portion sizes by measuring and weighing your food at meals for a couple of weeks. Eating too much carbohydrate at one time will elevate your blood glucose, even if the food is healthy.

4. Think about your appetite and what will best satisfy it. If you have budgeted 15 to 20 grams of carbohy-

drate for your bedtime snack, what would you rather have: 1/2 cup of ice cream (sugar free or not, it has about 15 to 20 grams of carbohydrate), a granola bar, or a medium-sized orange? The carbohydrate cost is the same; it's up to you to choose.

5. Purchase a carbohydrate counting book at any bookstore. The American Diabetes Association has published *The Diabetes Carbohydrate and Fat Gram Guide* by Lea Ann Holzmeister, RD, CDE. This book is helpful when you are eating a food that doesn't come with a nutrition facts label, such as many of our dinner foods or foods we eat in restaurants. The ADA has also published three booklets, at three levels of complexity, to use as a resource when you are learning carbohydrate counting: *Getting Started* (Level 1), *Moving On* (Level 2), and *Using Carbohydrate/ Insulin Ratios* (Level 3).

Other books to help you count carbohydrates are:

- *Exchange Lists for Meal Planning,* American Diabetes Association/The American Dietetic Association, 1995
- *The American Diabetes Association Guide to Healthy Restaurant Eating* by Hope S. Warshaw, American Diabetes Association, 1998

Commonly Asked Questions

Won't I gain weight if I expand my food choices and start eating foods that contain sugar? In most cases, health care providers do not assume that you are going to be able or willing to eat perfectly balanced meals and snacks every day. However, eating in the healthiest way possible is what is desirable for all people, with or without diabetes. It is now possible to live in the "real-food world" when you have diabetes. However, this does not mean that treat foods and desserts should be eaten in *addition* to all of your usual foods, but rather that they should be fit in, using a meal planning method such as carbohydrate counting, as part of the total carbohydrate allowance for a particular meal or snack.

What about protein and fat? Aren't they important anymore? We still want to help people meet the recommended guidelines for healthy eating. The amounts of protein and fat are still important, although they are not the main focus of carbohydrate counting and do not affect blood glucose as much as carbohydrate. If a dietitian notes that a person is adding high amounts of fat to meals and snacks, he or she may negotiate a certain number of fat servings to add per day. If weight loss is needed or decreasing cholesterol is a major goal, this will be taken into consideration. In addition, many Americans eat more protein in a day than the amount actually needed by their bodies. Therefore, most people are given a guideline that translates their protein intake into a certain number of ounces per meal.

What are examples of some common foods and their average carbohydrate contents? Some typical carbohydrate choices in common portions are counted as follows:

- Bagel, one large, 60–75 grams carbohydrate
- Banana, one large, 30 grams carbohydrate
- Orange juice, 1/2 cup (4 ounces), 15 grams carbohydrate
- Cornflakes, 1 1/2 cups, 30 grams carbohydrate
- Low-fat milk, 1 cup (8 ounces), 15 grams carbohydrate

- Fat-free yogurt sweetened with NutraSweet, 1 cup (8 ounces), 15 grams carbohydrate
- White or wheat bread, two slices, 30 grams carbohydrate
- Potato chips, one small bag, 15 grams carbohydrate
- Chicken noodle soup, 1 cup, 10 grams carbohydrate
- Ten jelly beans, 10 grams carbohydrate
- Spaghetti, 2 cups, 60 grams carbohydrate
- Macaroni and cheese, 1 cup, 48 grams carbohydrate
- Fried rice, 1 cup, 53 grams carbohydrate
- Corn, one medium ear, 19 grams carbohydrate
- Baked potato, one medium, 22 grams carbohydrate

Your Turn

Now it's your turn to recall some key points from this chapter. Let's see how you do!

1. The only "diet" that people with diabetes can follow to control their blood glucose and weight is the ADA exchange system. True or false?
2. You can only use carbohydrate counting if you are taking insulin. True or false?
3. When the body digests carbohydrate foods, about _____% is converted into blood glucose. Only _____% of protein and _____% of fat are converted into blood glucose.
4. It is more important to know how much carbohydrate you have budgeted for each meal or snack than to know your total carbohydrate allowance for the day. True or false?

See APPENDIX A for the answers.

8

Label Reading

James: I'm so confused. I just had my medical checkup last week, and my doctor told me I needed to lose weight and that my cholesterol was a bit high. Because I have gained weight over the past 6 months, my blood sugars have suffered as well. What numbers should I be looking for when I look at sugar and fat on food labels? I heard that if sugar or fat is listed in the first seven ingredients, the food should be avoided.

Dietitian: You are not the only one confused about what to focus on when reading a food label. Although most people look at food labels, it is impossible to interpret what the numbers mean without some education.

James: What about when a label claims the product is 'fat free'—is it really fat free? And what about 'low calorie'?

Dietitian: I can show you a quick and easy way to look at food labels and help you interpret the most meaningful information for weight and blood sugar control. By learning what items to focus on when reading a food label, you will find it easier and faster to read the label and to use your new knowledge to help you meet your particular needs.

James: I brought some food labels with me today, since these are some of the foods I use on a regular basis. I hope we can fit them all in.

Dietitian: Good idea. It is not necessary to give up your favorite foods as long as you know how to fit them into your meals or snacks. Let's get started.

What's Next?

Although we have read that the new food labels are easy to read and provide us with easy-to-use nutrition information, the labels are often overwhelming. With some nutrition education, James was amazed to learn just how quick and easy it was to read a food label and pick the foods that would help him meet his particular needs: weight loss, cholesterol control, and blood glucose management. Now, when he walks down the grocery store aisles and sees hundreds of food items, he no longer feels overwhelmed and restricted. He knows that a grocery list for a person with diabetes can contain a wide selection of tasty and nutritious foods—and that it includes the same foods that any healthy eater may buy.

The Old and the New

Nutrition labeling originally began in 1974 as a voluntary process for most foods. It was only required on products that added extra nutrients or made nutrition claims. Starting in 1994, food manufacturers had to revamp and update nutrition labels as a result of the federal government stepping in when food labeling got out of control during the deregulated 1980s. Labels had become confusing and untruthful, with manufacturers making meaningless health claims on their packaged foods.

The Nutrition Labeling and Education Act of 1990 required food packages to display the following new label format:

Nutrition Facts: This heading replaces the words "Nutrition Information" found on old labels.

Serving Size: This is found directly under Nutrition Facts and is the place to begin collecting needed information. "Serving Size" is probably the most important part of the food label because the nutrition information that follows is always given on a per serving basis. Serving sizes are now more uniform from one brand to another, making it easier to compare products. Manufacturers used to make their serving sizes very small to make their foods seem lower in calories, fat, and sodium and to imply that there were more servings per container. The serving size is now required to be in amounts that are closer to what most people actually eat.

Nutrients: Additions to the list of nutrients include saturated fat, cholesterol, dietary fiber, and sugars. These were added to the existing nutrients listed, total fat and total carbohydrate. The amount of the nutrients is expressed in two ways: as the amount by weight per serving and as a percentage of the Daily Value, which is a nutrition reference tool.

Percent Daily Value: These percentages are listed on the right side of the label across from the nutrients and can help you decide if a food contributes a little or a lot of a certain nutrient, without doing any calculations. They let you know how far a serving of the food goes toward helping you meet your daily nutrition requirements. (See "Daily Values" below.)

Vitamins and Minerals: Food labels were originally designed to provide more information about vitamins and minerals, since there were many deficiencies associated with the seven vitamins and minerals that had to be shown. Later, because few Americans are deficient in the three B vitamins—thiamin, riboflavin, and niacin—they were removed. However, these and others may be added if label claims note their presence in the product. Vitamins A and C and the minerals calcium and iron are still listed.

Daily Values: The list of daily values at the bottom of the label tells you how much of each kind of nutrient you need each day. The values listed for a 2,000-calorie diet are used to calculate the "Percent Daily Value" for each nutrient.

Ingredients: The ingredients are listed in descending order by weight. The sources of some of the ingredients, such as flavorings, must be identified by name in case they need to be avoided for health or religious reasons.

Here Are the Facts

Health Claims

Because of widespread fraud and potentially harmful health claims on food labels in the 1970s and 1980s, health claims linking specific foods with lowering our risks of certain diseases are now strictly regulated. The Food and Drug Administration (FDA) developed a policy that allowed only seven health claims to be stated, all of which have been supported by scientific evidence. These relationships that can be claimed on a label include:

1. calcium and a lower risk of osteoporosis (loss of bone mass)
2. sodium and an increased risk of hypertension (high blood pressure)
3. dietary fat and an increased risk of cancer
4. saturated fat and cholesterol and an increased risk of coronary heart disease
5. fruits and vegetables and a decreased risk of cancer
6. fruits, vegetables, and grain products that contain fiber, particularly soluble fiber, and a decreased risk of coronary heart disease

7. fiber-containing grain products, fruits, and vegetables and a decreased risk of cancer

Nutrient Content Claims

The new food labeling regulations also set strict definitions to address the problem of misleading nutrition claims. When you see a term like *low fat*, you can now believe it. There are only 11 nutrition terms that may be used, and these terms are strictly regulated to describe a food's nutrient content.

Free: Other words may be used in place of "free," such as *without, trivial or negligible source of, no, zero,* or *insignificant source of*. It is impossible to measure below a certain amount of a nutrient such as fat. So when a food label claims a food is free of fat, for example, it actually means that there is less than one-half gram (0.5 grams) per serving. Besides fat, free may also describe cholesterol, sodium, sugar, and calories.

Low or Very Low: Other words that may be used in place of "low" include *little, low source of,* and *contains a small amount of*. Low actually means that a person can eat a large amount of the food without exceeding the daily value for the nutrient. Low may describe total fat, saturated fat, cholesterol, sodium, or calories. The term *very low* may be used *only* to describe sodium.

Fewer, Less, and More: These terms are used when a regular product is compared to a nutritionally altered product. The comparison food must be identified, and although the foods don't have to be exactly the same, they do have to be within the same category. Take, for example, plain popcorn and potato chips. These are both snack foods, yet plain popcorn has "30% fewer calories" than potato chips. To use the "more" claim, the food must have at least 10% more of the daily value of a particular nutrient than the reference food; for example, whole-wheat crackers have "10% more fiber" than wheat crackers.

Light or Reduced: A "light," or "lite," or "reduced" product must have 25% less of a nutrient (for example, sugar, sodium, or fat) than a similar product (the original version) within the same category. For example, light ice cream must have at least 25% less fat or calories than regular ice cream, and reduced-fat cheese must have at least 25% less fat than regular cheese.

Lean or Extra Lean: These terms can only be used to describe the fat content of meat, poultry, seafood, or game meats. "Lean" foods have less than 10 grams of fat, less than 4 grams of saturated fat, and less than 95 milligrams of cholesterol per serving (about 3 ounces) and may include chicken without the skin. "Extra lean" means the food has less than 5 grams of fat, less than 2 grams of saturated fat, and less than 95 milligrams of cholesterol per serving (3–4 ounces) and may include fish such as cod or haddock.

High or Good Source: Other words that may be used in place of "high" include *rich in* and *excellent source*. The actual definition of high says that the food must have 20% or more of the daily value for that nutrient in a serving, while "good source" means that the food must have 10–19% of the daily value.

Common Terminology

Reading the food label can help you maintain and improve your health and, more specifically, your blood glucose control and weight—but only if you use it. To make the best food choices, you must be able to define the health claims as well as interpret the specific claims commonly used to describe specific nutrients. Here is a list of claims you will see:

- **Calorie free** = less than 5 calories per serving
- **Low calorie** = 40 calories or less per serving
- **Reduced calorie** = at least 25% fewer calories per serving than reference food
- **Sugar free** = less than 0.5 grams of sugar per serving
- **No sugar added** = processing and packing does not increase the sugar content over the amount naturally found in the ingredients
- **Reduced sugar** = 25% less sugar per serving than the reference food
- **Fat free** = less than 0.5 grams of fat per serving
- **Saturated fat free** = less than 0.5 grams of saturated fat per serving
- **Low saturated fat** = 1 gram or less of saturated fat per serving
- **Low fat** = 3 grams or less of fat per serving
- **Reduced or less fat** = 25% less fat per serving than reference food
- **Cholesterol free** = less than 2 milligrams of cholesterol and 2 grams or less of saturated fat per serving
- **Low cholesterol** = 20 milligrams or less of cholesterol and 2 grams or less of saturated fat per serving

- **Reduced or less cholesterol** = at least 25% less cholesterol and 2 grams or less of saturated fat per serving than reference food
- **High fiber** = 5 grams or more of fiber per serving and must also be low in fat
- **Good source of fiber** = between 2.5 and 4.9 grams of fiber per serving
- **Added fiber** = at least 2.5 grams more per serving than reference food
- **Sodium free** = less than 5 milligrams of sodium per serving
- **Very low sodium** = 35 milligrams or less of sodium per serving
- **Low sodium** = 140 milligrams or less of sodium per serving
- **Reduced sodium** = at least 25% less sodium per serving than the reference food

Here's What You Can Do

First, let's start by thinking of all foods as possible choices rather than putting them into the category "good" or "bad." Next, let's think about a quick and easy way to look at any food label, regardless of which aisle you are standing in.

Simply looking at a bunch of numbers does not necessarily translate into useful nutrition knowledge. When you read a food label, it is most important to be able to predict how the particular food will affect your blood glucose and your weight. To do this, it is helpful to have some easy-to-visualize reference foods to use for comparison so that you can interpret what you are eating in terms of familiar food items. The following guidelines will help you to accurately interpret any food label and to visualize its information. Take a look at the label from a granola bar, and follow the steps below.

Nutrition Facts

Serving Size 1 bar (28g)
Servings Per Container 10

Calories 120 Calories from Fat 35

	% Daily Value*
Total Fat 2 g	**3%**
Saturated Fat 0.5 g	**3%**
Cholesterol 0 mg	**0%**
Sodium 75 mg	**3%**
Total Carbohydrate 18 g	**6%**
Dietary Fiber 2 g	**5%**
Sugar 8 g	
Protein 2 g	

Vitamin A 0%	●	Vitamin C 0%
Calcium 0%	●	Iron 4%

*Percent Daily Values are based on a 2,000 calorie diet. Your daily values may be higher or lower depending onyour calorie needs:

	Calories:	2,000	2,500
Total Fat	Less than	65g	80g
Sat Fat	Less than	20g	25g
Cholesterol	Less than	300mg	300mg
Sodium	Less than	2,400mg	2,400mg
Total Carbohydrate		300g	300g
Dietary Fiber		25g	30g

Calories per gram:
Fat 9 * Carbohydrate 4 * Protein 4

Ingredients: Granola (rolled oats, whole wheat flakes, sugar,molasses, hydrogenated vegetable oils (canola oil and/or soybean oil). honey, salt, raisins, corn syrup solids, glycerin, almond pieces, coconut, whey powder, sorbitol, soy lecithin, cinnamon, natural and artificial flavor. May contain a trace of peanuts.

1. **Check the serving size.** Always start at the top of the label so that you won't miss any steps. Remember, although the serving sizes are now more uniform in similar categories of foods and are closer to the serving sizes that most people really eat, the serving size does not necessarily match the standard portion sizes on the *Exchange Lists for Meal Planning*. Also, you have to seriously consider how much you will *actually* eat compared to the serving size listed. If you eat more than the stated serving size, you will need to adjust all of the nutrient numbers accordingly. If the serving size looks ridiculously small, for example, "one cookie," you will have to ask yourself if you

are able to eat only one cookie and be satisfied. Maybe this product should be left on the shelf at the grocery store and not brought into your home. In the sample label, the actual serving size is *one granola bar* (the 28 grams listed next to the serving size is simply the weight of each bar).

2. **Check the total fat.** Working your way down from serving size, you'll notice total fat. This category will tell you immediately if this particular food is a good choice to decrease your risk of heart disease, cancer, and overweight. In the sample label, the total fat is 2 grams. Remember that 2 grams is the amount found in one bar. We can quickly glance just below to see how much of the total fat is coming from saturated fat.

   What does 2 grams of fat look like? To picture it, think of a pat of butter that you would receive at a restaurant. The little squares of butter that adhere to the cardboard backing are equal to 1 teaspoon of butter each. A pat of butter is also considered 1 serving of fat, and 1 serving of fat always has 5 grams of fat. So you can use a pat of butter as your reference food for 1 serving of fat. Now think of the teaspoon of butter being divided into five parts, one for each gram of fat. If you imagine coloring in two of the parts— 2 grams—you can visualize how much fat is in each granola bar.

3. **Check the total carbohydrate.** For a quick and easy label check, you are now down to the last nutrient, total car-

bohydrate. Looking at the sample label, you can see that one bar has 18 grams of total carbohydrate.

What does 18 grams of carbohydrate look like? To make the grams of carbohydrate more visual, think of a slice of bread. One slice of bread is an example of one serving of carbohydrate, and it is also easy for most people to visualize. One serving of carbohydrate is equal to about 15 grams. Because not all servings of carbohydrate foods have exactly 15 grams of carbohydrate, we can go up or down by 4 grams: 11–19 grams of carbohydrate will still be equivalent to one serving of carbohydrate. Think of a slice of bread as being divided into 15 parts, 1 for each gram of carbohydrate. In this case, you can imagine coloring in the whole slice to picture how much carbohydrate is in the granola bar.

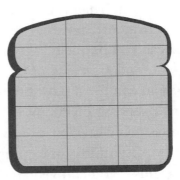

Putting It All Together

Let's review the information you have collected from the sample label:

- One granola bar has 2 grams of fat = less than one-half pat of butter

- One granola bar has 18 grams of carbohydrate = one slice of bread

Therefore, one granola bar will affect your blood glucose the same as if you had eaten one slice of bread with less than half a pat of butter on it.

More Things You Can Do

1. If you do not have an individualized meal plan, set up a meeting with a registered dietitian (RD) to determine the number of grams of carbohydrate and fat to aim for at each meal and snack.
2. Every time you read a food label, any label, ask yourself the following question: If I eat one serving of this food, how many pats of butter and slices of bread will the food be equivalent to?
3. Read, read, read. You will soon find out that you have been eliminating many foods that can easily fit into your meal plan. You will also begin to understand where some high blood glucose readings or extra pounds have come from.
4. Watch the serving size very carefully. Foods like peanut butter are fine when eaten according to the serving size, but they can be very high in fat and calories when portions are not moderated.
5. Compare no-sugar-added products with regular products. You will note that the carbohydrate content is often very similar. If the fat content is pretty much equal in both, then you can choose whichever product you want.
6. Watch out for fat-free foods. When fat is lowered or totally removed from foods, the sugar and/or starch is

usually increased to help stabilize structure and texture and enhance taste. Therefore, low-fat and fat-free foods are usually higher in carbohydrate. This does not mean that you need to avoid these foods—you just need to read the label carefully.

Commonly Asked Questions

Can I really believe it when a label says fat free? Yes, you can believe the claim. However, because it is impossible to measure below a certain amount of fat, the term fat free means only that there is less than 0.5 grams of fat *per one serving*. If you have a package of fat-free cookies and the serving size is one cookie, eating 10 cookies could mean eating almost 5 grams of fat.

Are serving sizes usually realistic? Serving sizes, for the most part, are now more standard within food categories, for example, frozen desserts such as ice cream and frozen yogurt. However, let's look at the common serving size for ice cream and frozen yogurt: It's only a level 1/2 cup! When is the last time you or anyone you know ate a level 1/2 cup of ice cream or frozen yogurt? The average person would likely eat 1 level cup of ice cream—or more—and would not agree that 1/2 cup is a realistic serving size. This reinforces the statement we made earlier that serving size is probably the most important part of the food label, since all of the nutrition information is always based on the serving size.

Why does the total carbohydrate always seem higher in fat-free and low-fat foods? When the fat is decreased or taken out of a product entirely, more sugar and/or starch is added to the product to maintain bulk, volume, texture, structure, moistness, and tenderness. Because this starch and/or sugar is added into the carbohydrate grams, these products are usually higher in total carbohydrate and have a greater effect on blood glucose. However, this does not necessarily cancel out the benefits of a low-fat or fat-free food.

Your Turn

Now it's your turn to recall some key points from this chapter. Let's see how you do!

1. Before the Nutrition Labeling and Education Act of 1990, some food labels were confusing, untruthful, and made meaningless health claims. True or false?
2. The _____ is probably the most important part of the whole food label.
3. If a bagel had 75 grams of total carbohydrate, it would be equivalent to eating _____ slices of bread.
4. If the nutrition label on a carton of ice cream lists 15 grams of total fat for a 1/2 cup serving, the fat in a serving would be equivalent to eating _____ pats of butter.

See APPENDIX A for the answers.

9

Weight Control

Denise: I think the reason I got diabetes in the first place is because I gained 20 pounds over the past 2 years.

Dietitian: Certainly gaining weight can put you at risk for developing type 2 diabetes, although there are other factors that are involved, such as family history.

Denise: Well, now that I have to take insulin, I find that it's a lot harder for me to lose weight than before I got diabetes. And my doctor wants me to lose 40 pounds! It will take me forever to lose that much weight.

Dietitian: Maybe trying to lose 40 pounds is unrealistic. The way to approach weight loss is to set small goals, such as losing just 5 pounds at a time.

M Y T H :

People with diabetes must be at ideal body weight to be healthy.

Denise: But won't it help my blood glucose if I lose as much weight as I can?

Dietitian: Actually, your blood glucose, along with your lipids and blood pressure will improve with even a 10-pound weight loss. Remember: every little bit counts.

The Old and the New

Before insulin was discovered, the only "treatment" for diabetes was to put a person on practically a starvation diet. The theory was that the less a person with diabetes ate, the less his or her blood glucose would increase. Unfortunately, this way of thinking has been applied to people who need to lose weight: the fewer calories a person takes in, the more weight he or she will lose. Although this is true, it has led to a multitude of starvation, fad diets over the years.

Remember the grapefruit diet? How about the cabbage soup diet? How about those medically supervised diets consisting of 800 calories per day? Sure, you lost the weight, but didn't it get harder to lose weight after a while? And here's the million-dollar question: how long did you keep the weight off? The medical community has learned a lot over the past few decades about the best way to lose weight and keep that weight off. The days of starvation regimens *should* be a thing of the past, since they don't work long term. Plus, many of these diets can be dangerous, particularly for people with medical conditions such as diabetes.

"Why bother to lose weight, then?" you may be asking yourself. "If diets don't work, I guess I'll just have to accept being fat." The good news is that first, you don't have to resign yourself to being overweight. Second, even a small amount of weight loss, such as 10 pounds, can be beneficial in helping you to manage your diabetes. Some people with type 2 diabetes are even able either to reduce their diabetes medication or to come off of it altogether with the right eating and exercise plan. (This doesn't apply to people with type 1 diabetes. They will always have to take insulin, although they may be able to reduce their amount if they are overweight and can lose some weight.)

Here Are the Facts

If you are overweight or have been in the past, you know more than anyone how those extra pounds affect your whole body. You probably get tired easily. You may become short of breath quickly. Your back, knees, or feet may hurt. You may even feel your heart pounding as you struggle to do the simplest chore. To make matters worse, if you have type 2 diabetes, being overweight makes it harder for your body to use its own insulin properly. If you continue to gain weight with diabetes, you may eventually find yourself on insulin. You may eventually develop high blood pressure and high lipid levels (cholesterol and triglycerides) as well. No wonder your doctor keeps urging you to lose weight!

The "Syndrome X" Files

Don't worry, we're not going to start telling tales of science fiction here. What we do want to do is explain a condition called *syndrome X*, sometimes called insulin-resistance syndrome or visceral-fat syndrome. Syndrome X and diabetes actually have something in common: insulin. To understand the concept behind syndrome X, or insulin resistance, let's review the role of insulin. Insulin is a hormone that helps move glucose from the bloodstream into cells for fuel. In people who are *resistant* to insulin, the glucose can't get into cells, no matter how much insulin is around. In fact, insulin levels in the blood often become high. This is the result of your pancreas producing more and more insulin in hopes that eventually those cells will smarten up, so to speak, and let the glucose in.

Why does someone become insulin resistant? In two words, *abdominal fat*. If you have a roll of fat around your middle (commonly called a "spare tire"), you have abdominal, or visceral, fat. This kind of fat is metabolically active: it constantly releases fatty acids into the bloodstream, which, in turn, makes muscle cells less sensitive to insulin. These fatty acids can also invade the liver, making it less efficient. The liver has a harder time breaking down insulin, and to make matters worse, it starts to release more glucose and more lipoproteins (particles that carry cholesterol) into the blood. And here we have syndrome X: too much insulin, too much glucose, and too many lipids in the blood, all a result of too much abdominal fat. Syndrome X can lead to diabetes, high blood pressure, and heart disease. Both preventing and treating syndrome X involve a healthful, low-fat eating plan as well as aerobic exercise.

Type 2 Diabetes

What if you already have diabetes? What's the weight connection? Most people with type 2 diabetes are overweight. They are usually advised to lose some, if not all, of the excess weight. Remember, with type 2 diabetes, your body may still be producing insulin. The problem is that your insulin doesn't work very well. If you are able to lose a few pounds, your insulin actually starts to work better because your cells become more receptive (or less resistant) to your insulin. This means that your insulin can now do a better job of controlling your blood glucose level. Another reason to lose weight if you have type 2 diabetes is that people with diabetes have twice the likelihood of developing heart disease. We know that being overweight increases your heart disease risk even further. Once again, the good news is that losing even 10–20 pounds can help accomplish all this.

Here's What You Can Do

Here are some tips that can help you lose a few pounds to help your diabetes (not to mention your cardiovascular system).

1. **Know your body mass index (BMI).** First, we want to introduce you to a concept called body mass index, or BMI for short. Now, before your eyes start to glaze over, realize that this is just another, but more accurate, way of figuring out your "fatness," so to speak. You might be familiar with the dreaded height and weight tables that insurance companies put out. Your doctor might even refer to a table such as this, all the while pointing out to you that, yes, you really should weigh 50 pounds less than you do, because the table says so. Many health professionals, however, don't like to use these tables (did we hear a sigh of relief

here?), because they are usually unrealistic. For example, how many men 5 feet, 6 inches tall do you know who weigh 133 pounds? If you do, hopefully they're not ill! We don't mean to totally put down these tables; they can be useful for reference. But we prefer to use BMI, and we think you will too.

BMI is a measure that adjusts weight for height, since weight alone doesn't really gauge whether a person is overweight or not. (Picture one of your favorite football players, for example; he may be "overweight" according to height-weight tables, but most of his weight is probably muscle.) Here's how you can calculate your BMI:

a. Multiply your weight in pounds by 703.
b. Divide the answer by your height in inches.
c. Divide again by your height in inches.

Let's do an example for someone whose height is 65 inches and whose weight is 190 pounds:

a. $190 \times 703 = 133{,}570$
b. $133{,}570 \div 65 = 2{,}054.923$
c. $2{,}054.923 \div 65 = 31.6$ (which rounds up to 32)

The National Institutes of Health (NIH) released new definitions of "overweight" and "obese" in June of 1998:

- BMI of 25–30 = overweight
- BMI of 30 or greater = obese

According to the definition, a BMI of 32 is obese, so the person in the example should take some measures to lose weight.

Although BMI is being used more and more by health professionals, the one thing it can't tell you is your percentage of body fat. This is something to consider when calculating and interpreting your BMI. Remember that solid, muscular football player? He may have a high BMI, maybe even putting him into the "obese" category, but most of his weight comes from muscle, not fat. On the other hand, someone may look slim and have a low BMI, but he may have more fat than muscle because he doesn't exercise. This person even has a higher risk of heart disease because of being more "fat" than "lean."

2. **Know your waist circumference.** The NIH also recommends that you know your waist circumference, which is linked to abdominal fat. All you need is a tape measure. Be sure to measure at the smallest section of your waist (abdomen) or just above the navel. Keep the measuring tape horizontal, and inhale and exhale once before you measure. If your waist measures more than 40 inches if you're a man or more than 35 inches if you're a woman, and your BMI is greater than 25, you have an increased risk for heart disease.

3. **Meet with a registered dietitian.** All people with diabetes are encouraged to meet with a registered dietitian to develop a *realistic* meal plan. A good meal plan not only can help you control your blood glucose, but it can help you lose and maintain weight as well. A meal plan should also provide you with a balance of foods and adequate nutrition. Maybe you've been handed a tear-off sheet for an 1,800-calorie "diet" by a well-meaning but busy doctor. This is okay just

to get you started, but it probably isn't realistic for you in the long run because it isn't individualized to reflect the way *you* eat and the foods *you* like. You need a plan, then, that you can follow long term. A dietitian will determine how many calories you need to lose weight safely. Your meal plan may consist of using the food guide pyramid, exchanges, carbohydrate-gram counting, or perhaps even fat-gram counting. There are many options for meal planning. You need to work with your dietitian to decide what's right for you.

4. **Learn to eat well.** Below are some guidelines that will help you make healthy food choices to help you lose weight without going hungry. If you constantly feel hungry when trying to lose weight, you probably aren't consuming enough calories, and therefore, your plan probably isn't realistic for you.

- **Use the power of the pyramid.** Your dietitian can show you how to use the food guide pyramid (see chapter 1) to be sure you consume the right amounts of foods and servings throughout the day. Most of your food choices should come from the "plant foods," such as grains, fruits, and vegetables. Fewer of your food choices should come from protein, milk, and fat. You should not eliminate any food group from your eating plan when you are trying to lose weight.
- **A calorie is a calorie is a calorie …** The bottom line for losing weight is to decrease your *total* caloric intake (while increasing your activity, of course). Carbohydrate and protein contain 4 calories per gram, whereas fat contains 9 calories per gram.

Obviously, it makes sense to decrease your fat intake because calories from fat quickly add up. But this doesn't mean you can expect to eat all the low-fat carbohydrate and protein foods you want either. Too many calories from any source can lead to weight gain. (By the way, alcohol contains 7 calories per gram, so you may want to go easy on alcoholic beverages.) A few words of caution about cutting calories, however: Women should not go below 1,200 calories a day and men should not go below 1,500 calories a day unless under medical supervision. Consider keeping a record of your food intake for a week or so, then bring it to your dietitian, who can help you determine how many calories you truly are consuming.

- **Focus on fat, first.** We know *all* calories count, but cutting back on fat first will automatically shave calories from your daily food intake. The first step to take is to reduce the amount of fat you add to foods with toppings such as butter or margarine, mayonnaise, oil, and salad dressings. You may decide to choose lower-fat or even fat-free versions of these condiments (but remember, they still contain calories). Second, reduce your intake of foods naturally high in fat: red meats, luncheon meats, cheese, whole milk, potato chips, ice cream. Your dietitian can give you a list of high-fat foods as well. Read nutrition labels for total fat. A food with no more than 3 grams of fat per serving is considered a low-fat food. Third, change how you cook. Bake, broil, poach, or grill your foods. Use cooking spray, broth, or water for sautéing or stir-frying.

- **Fill up on fiber.** High-fiber foods have the advantage of adding bulk; this means that you will feel more full. Foods high in fiber include whole-grain breads and cereals, fruits and vegetables, and legumes (dried beans and peas). Be sure to drink plenty of fluids when you increase your fiber intake to prevent constipation. (See chapter 3.)
- **Water works wonders.** You've heard it before, but water really can help you in your efforts to lose weight. No, you don't flush out calories or fat by drinking water, but water makes you feel full, contains no calories, and is a good substitute for snacking! Yes, you should try to drink at least eight 8-ounce glasses each day. Space it out over the course of a day and it won't seem like much. Plus, you can drink seltzer water, flavored or unflavored, or add your own lemon or lime to spruce up the flavor.
- **Get perspective on portions.** Maybe you eat all the "right" foods, but if your portions are too large, weight loss will be difficult. This is why you should dust off that food scale and dig out your measuring cups and spoons. Weigh and measure your foods for a while; you may be surprised at how much you're *really* eating. Practicing portion control at home will help you when you eat away from home, as well.
- **Eat six times a day.** What? Eat all day? How will you lose weight? Believe it or not, eating more frequently during the day can help in your efforts not only to lose weight, but to control your diabetes as well. Eating more frequently keeps your metabolism stimulated and keeps your blood glucose lev-

els more consistent. The key, however, is to eat *smaller* amounts of *lower-fat* foods; we're not talking six huge, fatty meals. Talk with your dietitian if you'd like to try this approach. (See chapter 12.)

5. **Change your behaviors.** One of the most difficult aspects of any weight-loss program is learning how to change the behaviors that perhaps led you to gain weight in the first place. Certainly, overeating and lack of exercise can pack on the pounds. But eating habits often become ingrained over the years, and they can be hard to change. The good news is that *any* habit can be broken and new ones can be formed. Maybe you tend to eat when watching television; if so, try eating only in the kitchen to break the association of watching TV with eating. Or perhaps you're an "emotional eater": you eat when you're upset, depressed, or simply bored. The key here is to find alternative activities to distract you from eating, such as writing in a journal, calling a friend, or going for a walk. You might even benefit from joining a support group. Keeping a record of when and why you eat can help pinpoint areas that you need to focus on.

6. **Become and stay active.** Exercise and activity are very important for anyone with diabetes. If you have type 2 diabetes, exercise will increase your sensitivity to insulin, which means that your blood glucose control will improve. Exercise lowers your risk for heart disease and cancer. Exercise helps to reduce stress. And of course, exercise is key if you are trying to lose weight. Why? Remember that exercise keeps your metabolism high. This means that you burn more

calories, even when you're relaxing. Exercise does this by increasing your lean muscle mass and decreasing your fat mass. Muscle burns calories; fat doesn't. As people age, they tend to put on 10 pounds of fat per decade! This also means that they are losing muscle. You can prevent this by becoming and staying active. Once you reach your weight goal, staying active will be extremely important for maintaining that weight loss. An exercise physiologist can help you put together an exercise program that is suited to you. (See chapter 13 to learn more about exercise.)

Commonly Asked Questions

My doctor said I need to lose 50 pounds to help my diabetes. How will I ever lose this much? If you are overweight, losing weight not only will help you improve your diabetes, but it will help you reduce your risk of other diseases as well. However, losing this much weight can seem overwhelming. Break down your 50 pounds into 5-pound increments; in other words, work on losing just 5 pounds at a time. Aim for losing no more than 1–2 pounds a week. And remember, losing even 10% of your weight will lead to health improvements.

I eat less now than I did when I was 25 years old, but I find I keep gradually gaining weight. What's going on? Unfortunately, you're experiencing what most people experience as they age: the 10 pounds per 10 years syndrome. Your metabolism has dropped, meaning that you just aren't burning calories like you used to. Make sure you're doing 30 minutes of activity at least five times a week. This will help boost your metabolism and, along with a healthful eating plan, will lead to weight loss.

I eat everything low-fat, I don't add fat to food, and I don't cook with any fat. I also walk four times a week. Why can't I lose weight? First, ask yourself how much you're eating of *any* food. You might be consuming only a small amount of fat during the day, but how much pasta or chicken are you eating? Large portions of any food can lead to weight gain, unless you're burning off those calories through exercise. Try weighing and measuring your portions, along with keeping a food record. This will help you see how much you're really eating. Second, sit down with a dietitian to work out a plan that will keep those portions under control. Finally, make sure you walk for at least 30 minutes, and consider adding some strength-training exercises to your routine to help build lean mass. An exercise physiologist can help you with this.

I can't seem to control my eating when I'm upset. All I want to do is devour a package of cookies. This is wreaking havoc with my diabetes, and I've been gaining weight. What can I do? Make a list of non–food-related activities you can do when you're upset, such as house cleaning, gardening, or another hobby. If possible, try not to keep tempting high-fat foods in your house. If you seem to be upset frequently, work on finding a solution to what is upsetting you in the first place. Maybe joining a support group or working with a therapist would be helpful.

Your Turn

Now it's your turn to recall some key points from this chapter. Let's see how you do!

1. Abdominal fat can lead to a condition called syndrome X. True or false?
2. You have to lose at least 30 pounds before your diabetes control will improve. True or false?
3. You must eat no more than 800 calories a day to lose weight. True or false?
4. List three steps *you* can take to help you lose weight:

   (1)_____

   (2)_____

   (3)_____
5. Calculate your BMI and measure your waist circumference.

   BMI: _____ Waist circumference: _____

See APPENDIX A for the answers.

10

Vitamin and Mineral Supplements

Cathy: I'm so confused! I don't know what to take. I read and hear about all these special vitamins and supplements that are supposed to be good for diabetes.

Dietitian: It certainly can be confusing for *anyone* these days, since there's more and more research coming out about what we really need to stay healthy and possibly prevent disease.

Cathy: Does this mean I have to swallow a handful of pills every day?

Dietitian: Not necessarily. The most important thing is that you're eating healthfully. In particular, you should be eating five servings of fruits and vegetables a day. If your eating isn't well-rounded,

MYTH:

People with diabetes need special vitamin and mineral supplements.

popping pills isn't going to help much. Foods contain many other substances that you just can't get in pill form.

Cathy: But I don't like certain foods, no matter how I try. Should I take *any* supplements?

Dietitian: That's a good question. Let's take a closer look at what you're eating and what you might need in the way of a supplement.

What's Next?

Can you identify with Cathy? The advent of the year 2000 has certainly brought a lot of changes, including changes in the way we think about food. Every day, researchers learn more and more about nutrition, especially about vitamins, minerals, and other types of supplements. Pick up a newspaper or magazine or simply turn on the television. There's sure to be a story about the latest vitamin you should be taking or food you should be eating more often. Walk down the aisle of any drugstore, or visit a health food store. The rows and rows of bottles are overwhelming. But what do we *really* need to eat and take to stay healthy and prevent disease? And do people with diabetes need special supplements?

The Old and the New

Chances are your parents or grandparents didn't take vitamin supplements when they were younger. Many supplements either hadn't been discovered or else not much was known about them. Today, ask almost anyone on the street if they take a supplement and chances are they'll say yes. The supplement industry is big business as well. According to the Center for Science in the Public Interest, a kind of "nutrition watchdog," so to speak, Americans spent $5.7 billion on supplements in 1997; that was up from $3 billion in 1990! In early 1998, *Prevention/NBC Today-Weekend Edition* conducted a survey to find out who was taking what and why. Here's what they found:

- 44% of Americans take a multivitamin
- 38% take separate supplements (i.e., extra vitamin C or E)
- 80% take supplements for good health
- 53% take supplements to prevent illness

On the flip side, the survey found that almost 40% of Americans don't take supplements. The various reasons included:

- They are unsure what to take
- They think supplements cost too much
- Their doctors don't recommend them
- They think supplements are unsafe
- They can get the nutrients they need from food alone

The last point is interesting: For many years people in the medical profession often scoffed at the idea that people needed to take supplements—unless there was a clear need for them, such as taking an iron supplement for anemia. They claimed that people should get all the nutrients they need from food (which isn't a bad idea).

Another reason for their skepticism, however, was that not a lot was known about what people should take, how much they should take, or possible harmful side effects of supplements. Today, we know more, even enough to start to make some concrete recommendations. In this chapter, we'll examine some of the more popular supplements and the pros and cons of each. One very important note: The information presented in this chapter is not meant to serve as medical advice; you should always discuss taking a supplement with your doctor or dietitian, since taking the wrong type or too much of any supplement may be harmful.

What Are Vitamin and Mineral Supplements and What Do They Do?

Let's first make sure you know what we mean when we casually chat about "vitamins, minerals, and dietary supplements." It always helps to define terms.

Vitamins come from living materials, such as plants and animals. Vitamins are needed in *very* small amounts to:

- process the food we eat
- help form blood cells
- help form DNA (genetic material)
- help form hormones
- assist enzymes in their various jobs

There are a total of 13 vitamins. They can be categorized as being either *water soluble* or *fat soluble*. Water-soluble vitamins are not stored in the body. These include the

B vitamins and vitamin C. Fat-soluble vitamins require fat to be absorbed and are stored in the body's fat tissue. These include vitamins A, D, E, and K. Although vitamins do not provide calories like carbohydrate, protein, and fat, they do help the body convert calories into fuel for energy. Vitamins often work in conjunction with minerals to maintain good health.

A *mineral* is an inorganic substance that is involved in numerous functions in the body, including:

- muscle contraction
- blood formation
- bone formation
- electrolyte balance
- nerve-impulse conduction
- energy production

Minerals are classified as being either *major*, meaning that they are found in the body in larger amounts, or *trace*. Major minerals include calcium, magnesium, potassium, phosphorus, chloride, sodium, and sulfur. Trace minerals are only needed in very small amounts. These include iron, zinc, chromium, copper, and iodine, to name just a few. Minerals work in balance with each other; therefore, a large intake of one mineral may interfere with the absorption of another and could result in a deficiency.

Dietary supplements include vitamins, minerals, amino acids, fatty acids, enzymes, fibers, herbs, steroids, and plant and animal substances (e.g., shark cartilage). The aisles of health food stores, drugstores, and even some grocery stores are brimming over with bottles of almost every supplement you could imagine taking. The question we need to ask is do we need these supplements and if so, which ones?

Most health professionals won't argue that a healthy lifestyle (eating right, exercising, not smoking, for example) wins hands-down over supplements any day. No vitamin will make up for eating high-fat foods, being overweight, or indulging in too much alcohol. Unfortunately, while many Americans know the basics of a healthful lifestyle, doing something about it doesn't always happen. For example, we need to eat at least 3 to 5 servings of fruits and vegetables every day, but the majority of us fall short of this recommendation.

Does this mean we should pop a vitamin to make up for the lack of nutrients? And what about disease prevention? Who *wouldn't* want to prevent cancer or heart disease by simply downing a pill with a glass of water once or twice a day? There are obviously several things you need to consider before you swallow that fistful of pills, including safety, effectiveness, and cost. The best way to find out what is right for *you* is to discuss this issue with your health care team before you make your decision.

The next few sections of this chapter are devoted to discussing a few of the main supplements that are discussed in connection with diabetes. Based on newer research concerning their role in health and disease prevention, they deserve a closer look. That's not to say that other supplements are *not* important, we just want to keep this chapter to less than a hundred pages!

Antioxidants

Antioxidants are substances that neutralize, or inactivate, free radicals. Free radicals are troublemakers. They are unstable oxygen molecules that damage cells, which in turn can lead to disease (cancer, heart disease, nerve disease, cataracts) and premature aging. These free radicals are formed from tobacco smoke, pollution, ultraviolet light, and X rays, as well as by our own body's metabolism. By neutralizing free radicals, antioxidants can prevent much of the damage caused by these harmful molecules. There are actually many antioxidants; some are vitamins, some are minerals, and some are even plant substances. Of the main ones—beta-carotene, vitamin C, and vitamin E—vitamins C and E are being looked at more closely in people with diabetes.

Vitamin C

Vitamin C is a water-soluble vitamin with known antioxidant effects. Some studies show that vitamin C can help fight heart attacks, strokes, cancer, and cataracts. There is some debate as to whether people really need to take vitamin C in the form of a supplement, since there are many foods rich in this vitamin. Eating several servings of fruits and vegetables each day can ensure that you're getting at *least* the RDA (Recommended Dietary Allowance), which is 60 milligrams (mg) for vitamin C. (A cup of broccoli has almost 100 mg of vitamin C.) Many people swear by this vitamin to prevent or lessen the severity of colds, and some studies show that it actually does help.

People with diabetes tend to have lower levels of vitamin C in their bodies, which may be due to higher blood sugar levels hampering the uptake of vitamin C into cells. A 1995 study that gave 2,000 mg of vitamin C to people with type 2 diabetes showed an improvement in both blood glucose and lipid (cholesterol and triglyceride) levels. However, more research needs to be done in the area of vitamin C and its role in glucose control.

- **Role:** maintains connective tissue; promotes wound healing; strengthens the immune system; may help to prevent cancer, heart disease, cataracts
- **Food sources:** citrus fruits, strawberries, cantaloupe, kiwi, red peppers, broccoli
- **Recommended daily amount:** at least 60 mg (currently being debated) from food or supplements
- **Possible harm:** more than 1,000 mg daily may cause kidney stones, diarrhea; stopping suddenly may cause rebound scurvy

Vitamin E

The evidence is strong concerning the role of vitamin E in the prevention of heart disease. Two important, large-scale studies out of Harvard found that men and women with the highest levels of vitamin E had one-third less heart disease than did those with the lowest vitamin E levels. Vitamin E has also been linked with preventing cataracts, cancer, and perhaps even Alzheimer's disease.

Recent research at the Joslin Diabetes Center in Boston, Mass., looked at the role of vitamin E in preventing and/or reversing kidney and eye damage. Results from this study suggest that vitamin E may reduce the risk of developing diabetic kidney or eye disease. However, it's too early to make definite conclusions or to know at what dose vitamin E exerts its beneficial effects. Other diabetes-related research has shown that vitamin E may help lower the level of LDL cholesterol, which is damaging to artery walls, and that it may reduce blood clotting in people with diabetes. At least two other studies have shown that people with diabetes who take vitamin E appear to have better blood glucose control than those who don't take vitamin E.

The RDA for vitamin E is 30 IU (international units), which is easily obtainable through nutrition or by taking a multivitamin pill. However, the antioxidant properties of vitamin E seem to kick in at doses of *at least* 100 IU and sometimes up to 800 IU. It's almost impossible to get this much vitamin E from food alone—unless you're willing to drink vegetable oil by the quart or swallow handfuls of sunflower seeds by the pound each day! For this reason, experts suggest taking a separate vitamin E supplement.

- **Role:** helps form red blood cells, muscle, and tissue; may lower the risk of heart disease, cancer, and Alzheimer's; may improve blood glucose control, arthritis, and immune function
- **Food sources:** sunflower seeds, wheat germ, vegetable oils
- **Recommended daily amount:** between 30 and 400 IU; for amounts above 100 IU, take as a separate supplement, ideally in the form of d-alpha tocopherol (better absorbed and used)
- **Possible harm:** amounts greater than 800 IU may increase the risk of stroke in people with high blood pressure; may interfere with medication that prevents blood clots

Minerals

Magnesium

There is a definite link between diabetes and magnesium: Magnesium helps the pancreas to secrete insulin. Inadequate magnesium means that not enough insulin is around to control blood glucose levels. Studies have shown that people who don't get enough magnesium in their diets have a higher risk of developing type 2 diabetes. In addition, a high percentage of people who already have type 2 diabetes have low magnesium levels, although it's hard to say which came first, the diabetes or the low magnesium levels. People with diabetes can lose magnesium in their urine if their blood glucose is poorly controlled. Diuretics (drugs for controlling blood pressure or fluid retention) can also leach magnesium from the body. Other people at risk for low magnesium include those who have congestive heart failure, heart attacks, diabetic ketoacidosis, or calcium or potassium deficiencies, and pregnant women. Magnesium may help prevent some of the complications associated with diabetes, such as eye disease and heart disease. However, no evidence shows that taking magnesium supplements improves blood glucose levels, since so many other factors are involved in blood glucose control.

- **Role:** involved with energy production; aids in muscle contraction, heartbeat regulation, and nerve transmission; needed for insulin secretion; may help prevent heart disease, stroke, osteoporosis, and migraines
- **Food sources:** whole-grain breads and cereals, legumes, nuts, bananas, green leafy vegetables
- **Recommended daily amount:** 320 mg for women; 420 mg for men
- **Possible harm:** large amounts may cause diarrhea, drowsiness, lethargy, impaired calcium absorption

Chromium

Chromium, in the form of chromium picolinate, has received a lot of press over the past few years thanks to claims that this trace mineral can reduce body fat and build muscle, all without dieting. No good evidence exists that chromium is effective as a weight-loss aid. However, chromium may play a role in the management of diabetes. Chromium is a trace mineral needed for metabolism and the production of glucose tolerance factor (GTF), which helps insulin to work efficiently. Several studies over the past 30 years have shown that chromium may help improve blood glucose and lipid (cholesterol and triglyceride) levels.

Unfortunately, it's difficult both to measure blood chromium levels reliably and to predict the response to chromium supplementation in people with diabetes. Researchers also do not know how much chromium we really need or how much is in the foods we eat, which makes it difficult to recommend a supplement dosage. Fortunately, this mineral is relatively safe, and the research thus far concerning chromium supplementation and diabetes control looks promising. In fact, many health care practitioners routinely recommend chromium supplementation for their patients with diabetes, especially those with type 2 diabetes. If you decide to try chromium as a supplement, first discuss it with your health care team. Don't take any more than 400 micrograms (mcg) per day, and be sure to check your blood glucose regularly.

- **Role:** aids in the metabolism of carbohydrate and fat; component of GTF, which helps insulin to move glucose into cells

- **Food sources:** brewer's yeast, whole-grain breads and cereals, orange juice, cheese
- **Recommended daily amount:** 50–200 mcg; up to 1,000 mcg with doctor's consent
- **Possible harm:** kidney damage and chromosome damage in extremely high amounts

Here's What You Can Do

Now you may be asking yourself: Do I need a supplement? If so, which one or ones? And how much? First of all, there are certain populations of people who may need supplements of one or more vitamins or minerals. Who are they and what might they need?

- **Women** may need calcium, iron, folic acid
- **Adolescents** may need calcium, iron, multivitamin/mineral
- **Seniors** may need multivitamin/mineral, calcium, vitamin D, vitamin B12
- **Vegetarians** may need calcium, vitamin D, iron, vitamin B12
- **Smokers** may need vitamin C

In fact, almost *anyone* could potentially benefit from a supplement if his or her diet is less than optimal. And with all the studies and reports coming out about how a particular vitamin may prevent a particular disease or condition, many people have started supplementing for this very reason. Below are some guidelines to help you make an informed decision:

1. **The first step.** Sit down with a dietitian. Do you skip meals? Dislike fruits and vegetables? Never drink milk? A dietitian is uniquely qualified to assess your current eating thoroughly, tell you what you're missing, and help you improve. Generally, the first and wisest step is to obtain any missing nutrients from food sources. If that's not possible, or if you're not willing, a dietitian may suggest either a multivitamin or an individual supplement.

2. **Where to begin?** Start with a multivitamin/mineral supplement. But even choosing this can be daunting! Your best bet is to pick a "multi" with no more than 100–150% of the daily value for the listed vitamins and minerals (there should be at least 20). Make sure it contains 400 mcg of folic acid and 400 IU of vitamin D. If you're a man, you may want to pick a supplement without iron because you require less iron than a woman.

3. **Additives, colors, and fillers ... oh my!** Unless you have a particular intolerance or allergy to a coloring or filler ingredient, such as lactose, don't worry about these ingredients. They may actually help with absorption. You'll simply pay more for a supplement without them.

4. **Store-brand vs. name-brand.** Compare the label of a store-brand multivitamin/mineral with the label of a leading brand. See any difference? Probably not. In fact, the only difference is—you guessed it—the price! Store-brand supplements are just as good as name-brand supplements (and may even be made by the name-brand manufacturer!) and cost less.

5. **Natural vs. synthetic.** In this day and age, anything that says "natural" has got to be better, right? Not

always, at least when it comes to vitamins and minerals. Natural and synthetic supplements are identical and will work in your body the same way. It's also less expensive to produce synthetic vitamins; therefore, you end up saving money. There's one exception: Natural vitamin E (d-alpha tocopherol) actually is better absorbed than its synthetic cousin, dl-alpha tocopherol.

6. **Healthy bones.** Unless you're either drinking at least four 8-ounce glasses of milk every day or eating about three 8-ounce containers of yogurt, you're probably short of calcium and should consider taking a supplement. Try to take your calcium in the form of calcium carbonate, which is highly concentrated. If you get gassy or become constipated, take a form called calcium citrate. Either way, take at least 1,000 mg of calcium every day (the amount of calcium in supplements will vary). Also, for better absorption, split your dosage over two or three meals, ideally taking no more than 500 mg at a time. If you rarely see the sun or are not drinking enough milk, take a calcium supplement with added vitamin D. Finally, choose a supplement with the letters "USP" on the label. This means that the supplement meets the U.S. Pharmacopeia's standards for dissolution.

7. **Antioxidants.** Taking antioxidants, such as vitamins C, E, and beta carotene, is more controversial than, say, taking a multivitamin. If you decide to take them, skip the beta-carotene (you should get this from food sources). Take up to 1,000 mg of vitamin C and up to 400 IU of vitamin E daily.

8. **With or without food?** Supplements are best taken with food, since they are better absorbed and will be available when the carbohydrate, protein, and fat are digested. The fat-soluble vitamins (A, D, E, and K) need some fat for absorption, so these should definitely be taken with food.

9. **Expired?** Supplements will lose their potency over time, so throw out any supplements past their expiration date. Also, keep your supplements away from heat, light, and moisture.

10. **Too much of a good thing?** Don't go overboard! Never take mega-doses of *any* supplement without first consulting your health care team. Use the guidelines mentioned above to help you. Vitamins and minerals can act like medications at higher doses and can be harmful.

11. **Other considerations.** If you are pregnant or elderly or have certain health or medical conditions (including diabetes!), please talk with your doctor *before* you take any supplement. And remember, *always* tell your doctor what you are taking at *every* appointment.

Summary

We hope this chapter has helped you sort out the often confusing world of supplements. As we learn more and more about supplements and nutrition in general, the guidelines above may change; this is inevitable when it comes to nutrition. This is why your health care team should be your partner in working to improve your eating and in deciding which, if any, dietary supplements you may need. Once again, remember that the ideal situation is to get your nutrients from food sources whenever possible. Eating according to the food guide pyramid (see chapter 1) will help you to make healthful food choices. Use vitamins and minerals for what they really are, supplements, not substitutes.

Your Turn

Now it's your turn to recall some key points from this chapter. Let's see how you do!

1. Vitamins and minerals contain calories and give us energy. True or false?
2. Antioxidants may help protect against certain diseases. True or false?
3. An example of an antioxidant is _____.
4. List two food sources of magnesium:

   (1) _____

   (2) _____

See APPENDIX A for the answers.

Sodium

11

Dietitian: How are things going with the meal plan we worked out last month?

Kevin: Pretty well, except that I think I'm eating too much sodium, and I know it's important to avoid using salt and eating salty foods.

Dietitian: You seem to be quite concerned about your sodium intake. Any particular reason?

Kevin: Well, I was told that people with diabetes can't have sodium in their diets. This has been hard for me, since foods don't taste the same without salt.

Dietitian: If you haven't been told by your physician that you need to restrict sodium because you have high blood pressure,

MYTH:

People with diabetes should always follow a low-sodium diet.

some sodium is okay. But if you do need to cut back on salt, there are ways to make food taste better using herbs and spices instead of salt.

What's Next?

Many people who have diabetes believe that they need to restrict their sodium intake, whether they have hypertension (high blood pressure) or not. The truth is, although some people probably should be careful of the amount of high-sodium foods they ingest, salt and sodium have nothing to do with blood glucose control. If you have diabetes and your health care provider has recommended that you watch your sodium intake, it's most likely because you either have high blood pressure or are prone to retaining fluid in your body, not because your blood glucose levels are running too high or too low.

The Old and the New

Mention the word "salt" or "sodium" to almost anyone these days, and he or she will likely tell you that *everyone* needs to follow a low-sodium diet. For years, health authorities, including the U.S. Department of Agriculture and the American Heart Association, have been informing us that we need to cut back on salt, since salt can raise blood pressure, which in turn, increases our chances of having a heart attack or a stroke. Researchers have been debating for decades about the role of salt in blood pressure control. For example, should everyone limit sodium intake or just people with high blood pressure? Does eating a high-sodium diet raise blood pressure and a low-sodium diet lower blood pressure? If a handful of people are what we call "salt sensitive," should we all cut down on sodium intake to be on the safe side? These are questions of extreme interest that even today are hot topics of conversation among the scientific community as well as at office coffee breaks.

As the twentieth century starts to wind down, a growing number of "salt skeptics" think that perhaps we've hyped up the sodium issue. Sure, most people with hypertension should probably limit their sodium intake, they concede, but maybe there are more important factors that control blood pressure. Some researchers will even go so far as to say that there is *no* good evidence linking a high sodium intake with high blood pressure. Furthermore, they argue, it's not necessary for *everyone* to limit their salt intake, since sodium has no effect on people with normal blood pressure.

What Is Sodium and Why Do We Need It?

We tend to use the terms "salt" and "sodium" interchangeably, but they are not really the same. Salt is actually a chemical made up of about 40% sodium and 60% chloride. Sodium is an essential mineral that we need to survive.

Sodium regulates blood pressure and blood volume and is important in the contraction of muscles and the conduction of nerve impulses. (Chloride, by the way, is another mineral that helps conduct the flow of water in and out of cells.) Sodium levels in our bodies are carefully and tightly controlled by the kidneys. Too much sodium in the body can cause fluid retention and too little sodium may lead to dehydration. Fortunately, our kidneys can get rid of any extra sodium that we take in, provided that they function properly.

Although most of us need to be careful not to take in too much sodium, some people, such as athletes or people who perspire heavily, need to make sure they take in enough sodium. Symptoms of sodium deficiency are muscle cramps, dizziness, exhaustion, and even convulsions and death. Luckily, it's pretty easy to replenish sodium stores: just eat some salty foods and drink enough fluids that don't contain caffeine.

Where Is Sodium Found?

Some amount of sodium is found in all foods. However, sodium that occurs naturally and salt added to foods at the dinner table are *not* the major sources of sodium in our diet. Most of the sodium in our foods is added during food processing. In fact, up to 4,000 milligrams of sodium that we ingest each day comes from processed foods. While some foods have an obvious salty taste—such as pretzels, pickles, and soy sauce, for example—you may be surprised to learn that some of your favorite foods may contain quite a lot of sodium, for example:

canned soup	luncheon meat	crackers
barbecue sauce	cheese	salad dressing
cereal	mustard	sausage
catsup		

Hidden sodium can be uncovered by reading the ingredient list on a food package. Here are some examples of high-sodium ingredients:

monosodium glutamate, or MSG (flavor enhancer)
sodium benzoate (preservative)
sodium caseinate (thickener and binder)
sodium citrate (controls acidity in soft drinks)
sodium nitrite (curing agent in processed meats)
sodium phosphate (emulsifier, stabilizer)
sodium proprionate (mold inhibitor)
sodium saccharin (artificial sweetener)
baking soda
baking powder

The Upside and Downside of Sodium

You've already learned about the importance of sodium in the body. Remember that this mineral helps regulate your blood pressure, muscle contraction, and transmission of nerve impulses. And when your body is functioning as it should, sodium keeps your fluid balance in control.

However, if you like to stay on top of the latest nutrition news, most likely you're well aware of the controversy surrounding the role of sodium in our diets, especially in relation to hypertension. It's often frustrating. To whom should we listen and what should we believe?

The Scoop on Salt

Most Americans like the taste of salty foods. Try eating unsalted potato chips or pretzels. Not so tasty, are they? And an ear of corn just isn't the same without a liberal shaking of salt. Yet while we may indulge ourselves in our passion for salty foods, we usually do so with a feeling of guilt: salt is bad for us, right? Sodium has been said to be associated with high blood pressure for a long time. Doctors and other health professionals usually advise their patients with high blood pressure to follow a low-sodium diet, often in conjunction with prescribing medications to control blood pressure. What is the connection?

A Blood Pressure Primer

Blood pressure refers to the force of blood pushing against artery walls as it flows through the body. Blood pressure can change many times over the course of the day and will go up if you're scared, upset, or exercising. Blood pressure tends to drop when you are relaxing or sleeping. When your blood pressure is measured, the reading will appear as two numbers. The first number, which is the higher of the two, is the *systolic* pressure. This is the peak force of blood as it is forced through your arteries by the pumping of your heart. The second number, the *diastolic* pressure, is the force of blood when your heart is relaxing between beats and filling up with blood for the next beat.

"Optimal" blood pressure is a reading of less than 120 over 80, usually written like a fraction: 120/80. A blood pressure reading of 140/90 is considered hypertension, or high blood pressure. People with blood pressure readings between 120/80 and 140/90 are thought to be at risk for developing high blood pressure. Blood pressure tends to rise as we get older.

Approximately 50 million people in the United States have high blood pressure (that's one in every five people). Almost half of the cases of high blood pressure are in people over age 60. In addition, high blood pressure is more common in African Americans and Hispanics and in people with diabetes, kidney problems, or a family history of high blood pressure. Other risk factors for high blood pressure include obesity, smoking, lack of exercise, and alcohol consumption.

High blood pressure is the most common of all the cardiovascular (heart) diseases. Untreated high blood pressure forces the heart to work consistently harder, leading to damage of the blood vessels, brain, eyes, and kidneys. It is the leading cause of stroke and one of the three main risk factors for having a heart attack (the other two are smoking and high blood cholesterol). So far, there is no cure for high blood pressure, but it can be controlled with medication and/or lifestyle changes.

The scary thing about high blood pressure is that there are few, if any, symptoms. More than half the people with high blood pressure do not even know they have it, giving this disease the label of "silent killer." Half a million people die each year from complications relating to high blood pressure. The economic cost of high blood pressure is an astounding $13 billion per year. While there are many ways to successfully manage high blood pressure, the unfortunate fact is that two out of three people do not receive treatment, and about 20% of people receive inadequate treatment.

What's the Connection?

How does sodium fit into all of this? Believe it or not, advice that people watch their sodium intake dates back to 2500 B.C., when Chinese physicians warned their patients to use less salt or else their "pulse" would harden. Since then, scientists have determined that the higher the salt intake of a population, the greater the incidence of high blood pressure. No one is exactly sure how sodium affects blood pressure, but it may be that too much salt in the diet damages sodium channels (which move sodium in and out of cells). Over time, the kidneys have a tougher time of trying to flush excess sodium out of the body, and blood pressure starts to climb.

Most of the information linking a high sodium intake to high blood pressure originates from 1988 data from the Intersalt Study. This study looked at approximately 10,000 men and women of all ages from different countries. The findings? First, researchers found that the higher the sodium intake, the higher the blood pressure. Also, blood pressure rose with increasing age in people from cultures that consume a high-sodium diet. The conclusion? A high-sodium diet causes high blood pressure. One problem with this study, however, is that it wasn't designed to show a cause-and-effect relationship; in other words, this was an observational study. The researchers did not intervene with the subjects' diets or lifestyle. They merely sat back, observed, and made their conclusions.

Because of this, you can imagine that the Intersalt Study has had its critics. For example, the Salt Institute claimed that the data linking salt intake and hypertension was weak, and that no good evidence shows that eating less sodium will improve blood pressure. Another study (funded by the company that makes Campbell's soup) showed that restricting salt intake did not affect blood pressure in most of the study subjects. However, this study's conclusions were based on analyzing about 56 out of 1,500 studies of blood pressure, a very small sample indeed. So small, in fact, that the researchers may have missed out on a larger percentage of studies showing just the opposite. In addition, there may have been some bias with this particular study, since a major soup company funded it.

The Intersalt Study researchers gave their study a second look in response to the criticism of their study methods. Once again, they concluded that there is a strong relationship between sodium intake and blood pressure, particularly in middle-aged people. This is not surprising, since we now know that blood pressure does increase with advancing age.

The bottom line is that cutting back on your sodium intake is helpful in decreasing and controlling blood pressure. This measure tends to help those who are "salt sensitive" more than those who are not (one out of four people with high blood pressure is salt sensitive). But since there is no laboratory test to determine who is and isn't salt sensitive, it seems prudent for all of us to go easy on our sodium intake, high blood pressure or not.

You can monitor your blood pressure at home and see for yourself how easing up on the salt affects you: If your blood pressure drops after following a lower-sodium diet for a while, you may be salt sensitive. Keep in mind, also, that you may have normal blood pressure now, but it's always possible that it will climb as you get older. The key, therefore, is to focus on *preventing* high blood pressure in the first place.

Other Problems with a High Sodium Intake

High blood pressure is the primary medical problem linked to a diet high in salt. However, there are other physical effects linked to a high sodium intake. For example, there is some evidence that a high-sodium diet can be a risk factor for osteoporosis, stomach cancer, and even asthma. So while you may have normal blood pressure, it may be prudent to go easy with that salt shaker to help keep your blood pressure normal and maybe prevent other serious health problems.

Here's What You Can Do

The evidence is there: In salt-sensitive individuals, salt can cause blood pressure to climb. The American Heart Association recommends that we limit our sodium intake to no more than 2,400 milligrams (mg) per day. This looks like 1 1/4 teaspoons of salt. Many health professionals will advise people with high blood pressure to cut back to 2,000 mg sodium per day. The average person consumes about 4,000 mg each day, or about two teaspoons of salt.

If you think you could stand to consume a little less sodium, here are a few things to consider: First of all, remember that sodium is found in all the foods that we eat. It's not wise or even possible to completely eliminate sodium from your diet (after all, it is an essential mineral!). Second, keep in mind that the *total* amount of sodium you ingest in your daily diet is important, not necessarily the sodium content of a specific food. This means that it's okay to eat a high-sodium food occasionally as long as the rest of your food intake is moderately low in sodium. Finally, the key to a healthy diet is to make gradual, small changes in your eating habits.

Rome wasn't built in a day, and it may not be feasible to stop eating all your favorite high-sodium foods overnight. If you're worried that foods will suddenly taste bland and dull, think about this: Studies show that people who reduce their sodium intake slowly over time adapt to a low-sodium diet to the point that low-sodium foods taste good and salty foods are too salty! By slowly making changes, you're less likely to notice differences in how foods taste, and the changes you do make will be permanent ones.

1. **Shake the salt.** One easy step you can take right now is to avoid adding salt to your foods, either in cooking or at the table. Start tasting your foods before you automatically add salt. You may be in the habit of reaching for the salt shaker before eating, so try not to keep the salt shaker on the table or even near the stove. Do you automatically sprinkle salt into the pan of water when you cook rice or pasta? Try leaving it out next time; the water will still boil. You can also limit or even leave out the salt called for in most

recipes. You'll never even miss it if you use other seasonings, such as black pepper, herbs, and spices. If you use packaged rice or pasta dishes, use only half of the seasoning packet; this can save you up to 500 mg sodium per serving. If you still feel you need to add some salt when cooking, add it toward the end so that the salt flavor won't cook away.

2. **Read nutrition labels on packages and containers of food.** The nutrition label on every packaged food must list the amount of sodium, in milligrams, contained in one serving of that food. Be sure to read the serving size because the amount listed as one serving may be a lot smaller than what you normally eat. In addition to the amount of sodium in one serving, the label will state what percentage of the recommended daily value of sodium (2,400 mg) is provided by one serving. Keep in mind that a food labeled "Reduced Sodium," "Unsalted," or "No Salt Added" can still contain a significant amount of sodium; these terms do not necessarily mean that the food is low in sodium. Take a look at chapter 8 to learn more about these terms and about how to read a nutrition label.

3. **Choose fresh, frozen, or canned foods without added salt.** Foods that are fresh or frozen (without added salt) are the best choices for you if you need to limit your sodium intake. Good examples are fresh fruits and vegetables; poultry, fish, and lean meats; and unprocessed whole-grain foods (breads, cereals, pasta, rice). If you use canned foods, buy those that say "no salt added" on the label or else empty the canned food into a colander and run it under

water to rinse away some of the sodium that it is packed in.

4. **Be careful when eating out.** If you eat out on a regular basis, you should be careful about your food choices in restaurants. Many dishes can be quite high in sodium. However, you can eat out and reduce your sodium intake by following a few simple guidelines:

- Once again, ignore the salt shaker on the table.
- Go easy on condiments, such as mustard, catsup, soy sauce, and salad dressings.
- Read menus carefully. Terms such as marinated, pickled, smoked, teriyaki, and "in broth" usually mean high sodium.
- Keep things simple. Foods that come with special sauces, gravies, or toppings are often high sodium. Order foods plain, if possible. If you wish to try a sauce or topping, ask that it be served on the side.
- Ask your server about any menu items you are uncertain about. Also, request that your foods be prepared without added salt.

5. **Use salt substitutes with caution.** Many people switch over to salt substitutes as an alternative to the salt shaker. Most of these "substitutes" contain potassium instead of sodium. The downside of these is that they often taste bitter. And there is a health concern: People with high blood pressure who take potassium-sparing medications should check with their doctor before using salt substitutes. They can be at risk of retaining too much potassium in their bodies, which can lead to heartbeat irregularities.

People with kidney problems need to heed this advice as well.

If you decide to use salt substitutes, keep in mind that some of them still contain sodium. It's important to read the label to be on the safe side. Remember, too, that you can always use seasoning products that have no sodium or potassium or make up your own mixture of herbs and spices to use in cooking and on foods.

6. **Check your medications.** Some medications, unfortunately, may contain sodium. Examples are antacids, headache remedies, laxatives, and sedatives. If you need to take any of these medications, talk to your doctor about lower-sodium alternatives.

Summary

Having diabetes does not mean that you automatically have to cut salt and sodium from your diet. However, you do need to limit your sodium intake if you have high blood pressure; if you have congestive heart failure; or if you are prone to retaining fluid. What if you have none of the above? Well, it's still a good idea not to go overboard with that salt shaker, particularly if it means you can keep your blood pressure down and possibly *prevent* high blood pressure from ever developing. Plus, a low- to moderately-low-sodium diet may help keep your bones healthy. If you think you could benefit from a lower-sodium diet, speak with a registered dietitian who can help you tailor an eating plan that's both palatable and healthful.

Your Turn

Now it's your turn to recall some key points from this chapter. Let's see how you do!

1. You should limit your sodium intake to no more than _____ mg per day.
2. Most of the sodium in our diets comes from the salt shaker. True or false?
3. Soy sauce is considered a low-sodium condiment. True or false?
4. List three ways that you can decrease your sodium intake over the next month:

   (1) _____

   (2) _____

   (3) _____

See APPENDIX A for the answers.

12

Snacks

Dena: What am I supposed to do? When I try to avoid snacking to keep my weight and blood glucose under control, I end up having low-blood-glucose reactions. Then, to treat my reaction, I always eat much more than I plan to eat—I just can't stop myself! If I try to snack between meals, I feel like I will never be able to lose weight because my snacks often end up being junk foods like chips, ice cream, and cookies—and I don't just eat a few!

Dietitian: To snack or not to snack? That is the same question those with and without diabetes always struggle with. Actually, snacking has many more benefits than drawbacks; however, *snacking smart* is the key.

MYTH:

People with diabetes should not eat snacks because snacking makes you gain weight and makes the blood glucose too high.

Dena: Does snacking smart mean only snacking when you feel a low-blood-sugar reaction coming on or when you are going to be exercising?

Dietitian: Actually, snacking smart means planning low-calorie, low-fat snacks every day, while at the same time not allowing your snacking to turn into another meal.

Dena: I know exactly what you mean. My dinner meal often goes on long after dinner, and most of the time I don't even enjoy the food and end up feeling guilty.

Dietitian: Well, today we can discuss why eating three meals a day with one or two snacks works better for eating healthfully, controlling weight, and maintaining blood glucose level, and also why planning your snack food choices will keep you from overeating at meals.

What's Next?

Like Dena, many people with diabetes struggle with the issue of snacking. Dena was receiving mixed messages about snacks. The first message was about weight loss: *If you want to lose weight, you have to cut down your calories and increase exercise.* The second message was about blood glucose control: *If you want to maintain control, you have to exercise, monitor your food intake, and yet snack between meals.*

In her attempt to stay healthy, Dena was trapped in a vicious cycle. The dietitian helped Dena understand that to maintain her weight, the calories she eats in a day must be equal to the calories she burns for energy in a day. When the calories are spread out over the whole day, within three meals and one or two snacks, it is *still* only the total amount of calories eaten in the day that counts. Rather than eating five or six times a day, Dena was eating only two or three times per day in an attempt to save calories. Unfortunately, the saved calories in the earlier part of the day were quickly "stolen" as treatment foods for low blood glucose or for food eaten at the dinner meal that never seemed to end.

Together, Dena and the dietitian devised a meal plan with healthy smart snacks that were planned for active and inactive days. This plan would help keep Dena's appetite under control and would provide adequate nutrients to keep her blood glucose stable between meals. Dena's meal plan incorporated three meals and two snacks per day while still allowing Dena to maintain her goal weight. Dena also learned why certain types of snacks sustained, or "carried," her appetite and blood glucose better than others. Once Dena understood how different foods affected her blood glucose, she was better able to eat well, exercise, and improve her diabetes control.

The Old and the New

Early in the twentieth century, eating and sharing food was a pleasant and important social experience. Food and meals were not continually related to concerns about health, dieting, and weight as they are today. Not only were people able to enjoy the "pleasures of the table," but they were used to more reasonable portions.

At the start of the century, before the modern conveniences, America's eating habits were typified by a three-meal pattern. Most meals were eaten at home, and working adults and children usually came home for the noon meal. Our ancestors took advantage of the daylight hours by rising at dawn to consume a large breakfast meal of grains, starches, proteins, and fat to provide energy for long hours of physical labor. They would return home to eat their large main meal, dinner, at noon before going back to more physical labor for the rest of the daylight hours. At the end of the day, they would eat supper, a light meal, before retiring for the night. Their meals were distributed throughout the daylight hours and snacking was not the norm.

Toward the middle of the twentieth century, foods began to be designed in quantities for people eating alone. The demand for convenient, ready-to-eat foods was on the rise. With the new food designs, we began developing a new pattern of eating called snacking, eating at any time or place. Our eating patterns began to include single-serving snack and convenience foods between meals. These foods were originally converted from our country's staple foods, such as potatoes and corn, but gradually more and more calories from fats and sugars were added.

Today, we no longer have time to eat the big breakfast and noon meal that our ancestors did. The noon meal is now only a short break in our workday. And large evening meals and nighttime snacks have become the norm. We eat fewer meals at home, and prepackaged foods, fast food, and take-out foods have replaced many of the pleasures of the table.

Here Are the Facts

Because we tend to associate snacking with junk food, the shared public opinion is that snacking is unhealthy. However, whether you have diabetes or not, snacking can be an important part of your overall healthy eating. For people who take insulin, snacks may be added into the meal plan to cover the time when injected insulin will be working its hardest and therefore prevent a possible hypoglycemic reaction. Hypoglycemia, a low blood glucose level, often occurs when a person on insulin or certain other diabetes medications delays or skips a meal or a snack. Eating regularly scheduled meals and snacks helps prevent this unpleasant experience. Snacks may also be added when you plan to be more active than usual, to provide extra fuel. However, for those who do not wish to snack, adjustments can be made to insulin or oral medications so that snacks are not necessary. For people with type 2 diabetes, snacks may help control appetite and prevent overeating at meals.

What Snacking Is Not

- **Snacking is not grazing.** A snack is a small amount of food eaten within a certain time frame, and it has a definite beginning and an end. Grazing is supposed to mean eating small amounts of food throughout the day; however, even though grazing may work for some people, this method usually results in an continuous eating binge without a planned beginning or end.

- **Snacking is not permission to skip a meal.** Snacks should be planned and eaten between meals, not in place of meals. This cuts down on real hunger, nibbling, and the risk of low blood glucose. If you try to avoid a snack or a meal to save calories and the result is a low blood glucose, you will end up eating many more calories than if you had eaten the snack or meal in the first place. Skipping meals only deprives your body of fuel and allows your body to assume it has to save rather than burn calories.
- **Snacking is not eating junk food.** Although we tend to think about candy, cookies, and chips as typical snack foods, snacks were never intended to be empty-calorie foods. Empty-calorie foods are the invention of our country's food suppliers and simply do not furnish wholesome nutrition in spite of all of the calories they add. Since junk foods take the place of more nutritious foods, try thinking of a snack as a mini-meal or any food that you would include in a meal but on a smaller scale.
- **Snacking is not a cause of weight gain.** Snacking between meals will only cause weight gain if you overeat at snack time. Weight gain often is the result of not snacking! For example, many Americans eat little if anything at breakfast, then a quick lunch only if there is time. Then they end up eating a huge amount of calories while waiting for dinner, at dinner, and after dinner, snacking continuously until they go to bed. So all of the calories saved during the day, and more, are quickly used up between 5:00 P.M. and bedtime! This common but harmful eating pattern denies your body of fuel in the early part of the day, while providing too much fuel at the end of the day. This leads the

fat cells to *store* more calories. When the food is spread out more evenly throughout the day, your body is better able to *burn* more calories.

- **Snacking is not eating in your car or at your desk or in front of the TV set.** Snacking works best when you don't associate snack foods with too many different areas of your house and life. When you eat a snack, try to sit down and enjoy it, even if you only have 5 minutes to eat it. Remember, the most important thing to think about is location, location, location.

- **Snacking is not keeping junk food in the house.** Snacking is keeping your surroundings junk-food-free for the most part. Only keep planned, healthy snacks in plain view at home or at work. And only eat these snacks at a fairly consistent time each day. This does not mean that you can never eat so-called junk food. Save it for special occasions, such as visiting friends, attending office parties, or celebrating holidays, or just for one of those days when nothing else will do. Better yet, *plan* 2 or 3 days during the week when you will allow yourself one of your favorite junk foods at a snack. Buy that food only in single servings. That way it is easier to plan the quantity so that you don't overeat. For instance, buy small, single-serving-size bags of chips instead of a large family-size bag.

- **Snacking is not being hungry.** Snacking allows an even flow of fuel (calories) to the body, at planned intervals of roughly every 3–4 hours. This should allow most people to begin identifying the normal signals of hunger rather than eating unconsciously out of boredom or stress. We all can become more aware of why, when, and what we are eating between meals if we do not create real hunger pangs.

Here's What You Can Do

Food suppliers have become more sensitive to our need for more healthy snacks. Not only are we being provided with a variety of healthy snack choices, but these choices are now available in single-serving sizes. Even cookies and chips are offered with less fat and calories—assuming that we eat only what the serving size indicates and not the whole package. Below are some tips to help you turn your grazing into planned snacking and choose the best foods for snacking smart.

1. **Plan your snacks.** Visit with a registered dietitian to help plan your meals and snacks on a meal plan that will work with your home and work schedules. If your meal/snack schedule is written on a meal plan and in plain sight, it is more likely that your timing will become routine. When you know that your food intake is planned for every 3–4 hours, you will become less anxious waiting for the next meal or snack. Try to stay within a half-hour on either side of your planned meal- or snack-time. For example, if you plan your snack for 3:30 P.M., you can eat it anytime between 3:00 and 4:00 P.M.

2. **Keep a written food record to get started.** To better estimate when and where your snacking goes off track, keep a food record for 1 week, including the weekend. This record should include:

   - the timing of your meals and snacks, or WHEN
   - the actual foods you eat and drink at meals and snacks, or WHAT
   - the amount of the foods eaten, or HOW MUCH

- the reason you are eating (snack-time, boredom, stress), or WHY
- the location at which you are eating (car, desk, in front of the TV), or WHERE

Keeping an honest food record will help you troubleshoot problem areas. This record will help you to answer the following six questions:

- Is your food evenly spread out over the day?
- What interferes with your ability to eat consistent snacks?
- When and where do you tend to overeat?
- Are regular snacks helping you to eat smaller meals?
- Have the snacks helped to regulate your blood glucose?
- Have you cut down the number of junk food snacks you are eating?

3. **Choose long-lasting snacks.** A snack with staying power (like a mini-meal) is usually one with some carbohydrate combined with a small amount of protein and fat. To give you some ideas, the items in Table 1 can be mixed and matched or maybe even doubled to meet your snack needs as indicated on your meal plan and to provide healthy, long-lasting snacks.

Commonly Asked Questions

What about my bedtime snack—shouldn't I omit it so that my blood glucose will not be high in the morning?

TABLE 1

One Carbohydrate (each of these foods contains about 15 grams of carbohydrate)	One Protein (each of these foods contains about 7 grams of protein)
1 slice of bread	1 ounce low-fat cheese
1/2 English muffin	1 level Tbsp. peanut butter
Half a 2-ounce bagel	1/4 cup low-fat ricotta cheese
Half a 6-inch pita bread	1/4 cup tuna
2 plain rice or popcorn cakes	1/4 cup low-fat cottage cheese
2 pretzel rods	1 ounce low-fat luncheon meat
5 melba toasts	2 Tbsp. grated cheese
3 cups low-fat popcorn	1 low-fat hot dog
6 saltine crackers	1 hard-boiled egg
8 ounces fat-free or low-fat milk*	
8 ounces plain yogurt*	

* Counts as one carbohydrate plus one protein

A bedtime snack is probably the most important snack of the day, especially if you are taking insulin or a diabetes pill that lowers your blood glucose. Your body still uses some fuel while you are sleeping. To ensure that your blood glucose does not drop in the middle of the night, possibly because of an active day or unplanned exercise, your bedtime snack could contain up to 20 to 30 grams of carbohydrate and possibly a small amount of protein and fat. If you have had an inactive day, a snack with 15 grams of carbohydrate may be enough.

Do you mean that I can have *any* snack that contains about 15 grams of carbohydrate, as long as it is low in fat? The main concern for anyone who eats snacks, whether he or she has diabetes or not, is always snacking smart. This means eating nutritious snacks that are high in fiber and low in fat; for example, a piece of fruit or some whole-grain crackers. However, it is still important to allow yourself a treat once in a while, as long as you stay within your carbohydrate allowance.

I'm still not sure whether I need two or three snacks a day. I have a hectic work schedule and often have low-blood-glucose reactions. How do I know how many snacks I need to eat? An appointment with a registered dietitian will help you determine what will work best for you. The dietitian will consider factors such as the timing and types of your regular meals, your activity level, your work schedule, your insulin or diabetes pills, and your weight goals. More importantly, the dietitian will take into account whether snacks are desired or needed to meet your personal diabetes management goals.

Your Turn

Now it's your turn to recall some key points from this chapter. Let's see how you do!

1. For people who take insulin, snacks may be added into the meal plan to cover the times when insulin is working its hardest. Additional snacks may be added when you plan to _____.
2. For those with type 2 diabetes, snacks may help control the _____ and prevent overeating at _____.

3. List three things snacking is not:

(1)_____

(2)_____

(3)_____

If you are trying to lose weight, you must give up snacking. True or false?

See APPENDIX A for the answers.

13

Exercise

Robert: I know exercise is important for me to stay at a healthy weight and to manage my blood glucose, but I'm having a hard time trying to fit it in every day.

Dietitian: It certainly can be difficult to exercise every day, given our busy schedules and lifestyles. And while regular exercise is important for good diabetes control, you don't have to exercise every day to reap the benefits.

Robert: I guess I thought I had to do some form of exercise every day, like walking or biking, and I get discouraged when I just don't have time.

Dietitian: Fitting in *some* physical activity each day is ideal, whether you actually

M Y T H :

People with diabetes must exercise every day to stay healthy.

167

exercise or do yard work or even climb the stairs in your house or office building. *Any* physical activity that you do daily will help keep you fit, help your cardiovascular system, and keep your blood glucose down.

Robert: So it's possible for everyone to stay active without having to become an athlete, and it's also possible to fit something in each day. Every little bit that I do is only going to help my blood glucose stay under better control.

The Old and the New

Mention the word exercise and chances are, if you're like most people, you probably think of sore muscles, heavy breathing, sweating ... not to mention the difficulty of fitting it in to your daily schedule. For many people, exercise is connected to a negative image, ranging from having to run around the track in grade school, to being stuck (literally) out in left field, to sharing an aerobics class with "twentysomethings" in spandex while the instructor screams orders like a drill sergeant. Maybe you had an unpleasant experience during your last attempt at exercise. Perhaps you went out and bought expensive running shoes and running clothes, then ran as fast as you could around the block, only to return home gasping for breath and limping, barely able to walk the next day.

If this sounds familiar, don't despair. The meaning of exercise has greatly changed since grade school and even since the aerobics craze of the 1980s (remember "no pain, no gain"?). Would you believe that climbing a flight or two of stairs in your office, playing a game of Frisbee with your kids, gardening, or mopping the kitchen floor can give you some of the same benefits as jogging, biking, or skiing? No? Well, read on!

Here Are the Facts

Surprisingly, only 22% of adults in the United States are regularly active. Yet, we know exercise is good for us. We know that it reduces our risk of heart disease and has many other health benefits. We've been hearing this for years. What many people may not know, however, is that 30 minutes of moderate exercise (physical activities such as walking or dancing) can be just as effective in disease prevention as the same amount of time spent doing strenuous exercise. In other words, you don't need to sweat in a gym for 30 minutes every day to be healthy, but you do need to try to accumulate 30 minutes of physical activity every day. If you don't think you can do all 30 minutes at one time, break your activity into two or three blocks of time, such as three 10-minute walks.

Benefits of Physical Activity for Diabetes

You may already have diabetes, but you may want to share the following information with family and friends, particularly if they are at risk of developing diabetes. Good evidence suggests that active people are less likely to develop type 2 diabetes than inactive people. As you know, having diabetes means that you have difficulty managing the glucose circulating in your bloodstream. If you have type 2 diabetes, your cells may be "insensitive" to insulin, meaning that glucose has difficulty entering cells. When levels of glucose stay high in the blood for long periods of time, complications of diabetes can occur, such as kidney and nerve damage, and eye problems. Many people who are at risk for developing diabetes also have high insulin levels in their blood, which can increase the risk for heart disease. Weight loss is effective in lowering both blood glucose and blood insulin levels, but physical activity may be even more effective in increasing insulin sensitivity, thereby lowering blood glucose levels.

If you have diabetes, physical activity, along with a healthy eating plan, can help you lower your blood glucose and gain better blood glucose control. You may even be fortunate enough to reduce the amount of diabetes medication you take, or even get off your medication completely! (Never change the amount of your diabetes medication or stop taking your medication without discussing this with your doctor first.) The key, however, is making physical activity a regular part of your routine.

Benefits of Physical Activity for Weight Control

Physical activity is a key factor in any weight reduction and weight maintenance program. It can supplement a reduced-calorie eating plan and help you achieve your weight-loss goals. But how?

Muscle is really the only tissue in the body that burns calories, and we use muscles to do just about everything, ranging from yawning, to writing a letter, to ice skating in the park. Muscles are constantly being broken down and rebuilt. Fat, on the other hand, is *much* less active than muscle. It burns hardly any calories. Fat deposits itself in fat cells and sits there until called upon as a reserve form of fuel. Our bodies easily accumulate fat and lose muscle if we're not physically active. This translates into a slower metabolism and ultimately weight gain. Physical activity helps you build and maintain muscle mass. And the more muscle mass you have, the more calories you will burn, even when you're relaxing. So physical activity helps with weight loss and maintenance in two ways:

1. by burning calories
2. by building muscle, which burns calories

Here's What You Can Do

It's never too late to become more physically active. You don't have to become a bodybuilder or go to the gym to pump iron. You will, however, need to get in some kind of physical activity every day and add regular aerobic and muscle strengthening exercises a few times a week to keep your metabolism burning steady and your risk from disease low. Here's what you will ultimately need to do:

- 30 minutes of physical activity every day (anything that gets you moving!), including
- an aerobic activity at least three times a week
- strength training two or three times a week

Aerobic Exercise

Aerobic exercise helps get oxygen to your heart, which then helps get oxygen to your muscles. Your muscles can then use oxygen to produce energy. Aerobic exercise can burn anywhere from 200 to 400 calories per 30 minutes, depending on the type of exercise you are doing. For example, running will burn more calories in 30 minutes than walking for 30 minutes because the intensity of running is harder than walking. This doesn't mean, however, that you have to start running. Walking is an effective, safe, and easy activity that will give you many of the same benefits as more strenuous forms of exercise.

Other interesting benefits of aerobic exercise are that it often helps to reduce your appetite so that you consume fewer calories and that it will help keep your metabolism elevated several hours after you stop exercising. What are some examples of aerobic activities?

- walking
- jogging
- jumping rope
- swimming
- dancing
- ice skating
- biking
- cross-country or downhill skiing
- playing sports such as basketball or tennis
- mowing the lawn
- raking leaves

You should aim to do some type of aerobic activity at least three times a week for a continuous 20–30 minutes.

If you choose to garden, do housework, or do yard work as your form of aerobic activity, the intensity should be about the same as going for a brisk walk.

Strength Training

Strength training both prevents loss of muscle mass and helps to build muscle mass. It's important to include some type of muscle-strengthening activities in your routine to supplement your aerobic activities. Don't worry—you won't end up with bulging muscles if you don't want them. But you *will* have better muscle tone and more strength to help you perform everyday activities such as carrying groceries or climbing stairs. Strength training *can* take the form of weight lifting, with dumbbells or barbells, or going to a health club and using the weight equipment. But it can also come from doing calisthenics, such as sit-ups and leg lifts. You don't have to have a set of barbells either. How about using cans of soup or plastic jugs filled with water? Whatever you choose to do to build lean body mass, you should aim for doing it at least twice a week. However, you should not do the same strength training exercises every day—you need a rest day in between to help your muscles recover.

Some people dismiss the idea of strength training because of health or medical problems or because they think they're too old. But almost anyone can do some form of strength training. Of course, you must get your doctor's consent before starting *any* exercise program, but strength training can actually help increase bone mass, help people with arthritis move more freely, help prevent stiffness, make you stronger, and of course, help with weight loss. Pretty amazing!

Getting Started with Exercise

It is beyond the scope of this chapter to give you specific activities and training tips. If you've already increased your level of day-to-day physical activity (e.g., walking for 30 minutes every day) and are ready to try something more strenuous, we recommend you consult with an exercise physiologist, preferably one who is also a certified diabetes educator. An exercise physiologist can prescribe an exercise program that is right for YOU and that will take into account any health or medical problems. This is very important, especially if you are considerably overweight or have high blood pressure, heart disease, arthritis, or diabetes-related complications such as neuropathy, retinopathy, or nephropathy. Don't assume that the trainer at your local health club is qualified; he or she may not have the proper education and training. Ask your health care team about scheduling an appointment with an exercise physiologist if you have not been exercising and would like to start.

In addition to learning how to exercise safely and properly, it's important to discuss your plans with your doctor before you get started. Your doctor may recommend only certain types of exercise for you, especially if you have any medical complications. Specifically, notify your doctor before starting exercise if you:

- have high blood pressure
- have chest pains or have had a heart attack
- have irregular heartbeats
- have more than 20 pounds to lose
- are short of breath after mild exertion
- have wounds or cuts that don't seem to heal

- have pain in your calves, thighs, or buttocks when walking
- have retinopathy (eye disease)
- have neuropathy (nerve damage)
- have nephropathy (kidney damage)
- have uncontrolled blood glucose

Phew! We know that's a long list. The good news is that even if you experience some of the above situations, you can probably still do *some* kind of physical activity. Some forms of activity are better than others for certain conditions. For example, people with retinopathy probably shouldn't do activities that involve heavy lifting or straining. This doesn't mean, however, that they can't use an exercise bike or a treadmill. So you see, it's very important that you find out what is right for you.

Commonly Asked Questions

What about hypoglycemia? If you have type 2 diabetes and manage it through diet and exercise, you will not experience hypoglycemia. Also, there are certain diabetes medications that do not cause hypoglycemia. It's important to find out from your health care team if your particular diabetes medication can cause hypoglycemia and, of course, how to treat it.

If you're already physically active and take insulin or certain oral diabetes medications, you probably know by now that exercise usually causes your blood glucose to drop, sometimes to the point where it drops *too* low and you then need to treat that low blood glucose (hypoglycemia). Exercise helps you use your insulin more efficiently to move glucose from your bloodstream into your cells, thus helping keep the glucose in your blood at a normal level. But if you exercise when your medication or insulin is peaking (working its hardest), you may experience a low blood glucose. A low blood glucose can also occur during exercise if you have not eaten enough or if it's been a few hours since your last meal, if you exercise for a longer time than usual, or if you exercise harder than usual. Other factors, such as the temperature, the humidity, and the weather conditions (if outside), can play a role. Remember, you may have a low blood glucose during or after exercise. You may even have a low blood glucose *hours later*. This happens because your muscles are replenishing their stores of glucose by taking glucose from your bloodstream.

Always be sure to carry some form of fast-acting carbohydrate (such as glucose tablets, a tube of instant glucose, or a box of juice) with you whenever you exercise, along with identification stating you have diabetes. You can limit your chances of having exercise-related hypoglycemia by doing a few things:

- **Adjusting your insulin.** If you take insulin, talk to your health care team about learning how to adjust your insulin, if necessary, to prevent going low. For example, if you take an intermediate-acting insulin, such as NPH or lente, in the morning, and you want to exercise before supper, when this insulin is peaking, you might take fewer units than you normally would in the morning. Or if you take a quicker-acting insulin, such as regular or lispro, and you plan to exercise after supper, you might decrease your supper dose by a few units. Your health care team can even help you with adjusting insulin if you're going to be active for extended periods of time (when skiing or hiking, for example).

- **Adjusting your medication.** If you take oral diabetes medication, it is important that you *do not* make adjustments in the dosage without first discussing this with your health care team. However, with regular exercise and activity, you may be able to reduce your dose and perhaps even eliminate the need for medication altogether.

- **Adjusting your food intake.** If your exercise or activity is unplanned and you've already taken your medication or insulin, if you don't feel comfortable adjusting your insulin, or if you expect to be exercising strenuously, it's a good idea to make some changes in your eating plan. For example, if you are exercising after a meal, you may want to increase your carbohydrate intake at that meal by 15–30 grams. Or, if you exercise between meals, it may be a good idea to take a snack of 15–30 grams of carbohydrate beforehand, such as a piece of fruit, a granola bar, or some peanut butter crackers. You must also take into account your blood glucose reading *before* you begin to exercise. Checking your blood glucose is crucial. Your dietitian or exercise physiologist can give you more food adjustment guidelines.

What about hyperglycemia? Believe it or not, physical activity can actually have the *reverse* effect on your blood glucose: it can raise it. When you start to exercise, your liver releases glucose to make sure that your muscles have enough fuel, no matter what your blood glucose level may be. If you exercise when your blood glucose is on the high side, exercise can make your blood glucose go even higher. For people with type 1 diabetes, this can be a potentially dangerous situation. When you are lacking insulin and have high blood glucose, you run the risk of developing ketoacidosis, which is very serious and can be life-threatening if not treated quickly.

For this reason, we recommend that you *not* do physical activity when your blood glucose is above 250 mg/dl unless you are in good diabetes control. If your blood glucose is higher than 250 but under 300, try exercising. If your blood glucose increases, stop exercising and call your health care team. If you have type 1 diabetes, you should always check for ketones when your blood glucose is above 250. If you have ketones, do not exercise. (Your health care team can show you how to check for ketones if you do not know how.) If you have type 2 diabetes, you will not form ketones, but you should not exercise if your blood glucose is above 300.

How do I stay motivated to be physically active? People who don't exercise usually have a list of reasons why they can't exercise. Often it's "I just don't have time" or "Joining a health club is too expensive." Look past these excuses and what you'll see is a person who is perhaps afraid or hesitant about "just doing it." Most likely this person also feels guilty because he is *not* exercising and knows he should. Here are a few tips for you to think about if you are one of these people—maybe you'll change your mind:

■ Consult your health care provider to make sure it's safe for you to exercise. Then, try to meet with an exercise physiologist to develop a program that works for *you*, not for your next-door neighbor.

- Wear comfortable workout clothes that fit. Also, invest in a good pair of sneakers that are appropriate for what you'll be doing.

- Don't do too much at once even when the temptation is there. Start with 5 or 10 minutes of activity if that's what you can do comfortably. You'll quickly build up. Take it slowly.

- Schedule an "appointment" for activity. Treat your exercise sessions just like your other appointments. Write them in your date book or on your calendar. By doing this, you're treating exercise as a priority.

- Enlist the support of family or friends. If time truly is an issue for you, maybe your spouse would be willing to get the kids off to school a few mornings a week so that you can exercise then, for example.

- Do an activity with a family member or a friend. That way, if you're not in the mood, your companion will be there to talk you out of skipping your workout.

- Or do it alone. Some people find they do better when they are on their own. For them, exercise is time to focus and reflect on the day or on important matters.

- Do something you enjoy. If you hate the exercise bike, you'll come up with 101 excuses not to use it. Ask yourself what you would like to do, or at least, what you'd tolerate doing. Perhaps walking or swimming appeals more to you.

- Still bored with usual types of exercise? Try something new, like tai chi. Or do something you might not even think of as exercise, such as swing dancing or country line dancing lessons. Besides having fun and meeting new people, you'll get a great workout.

- Vary your routine. Walking the same route day in and day out can get boring. Try a new route. Or try a different activity altogether. Not only does this add variety, but also different activities work different muscles, so you'll end up with a more thorough exercise plan.

- Exercise to music. Music that is upbeat and uplifting often helps you soar through your workout. Or, watch the news or your favorite TV show while you're exercising to help pass the time. Some types of exercise equipment, such as treadmills and stationary bikes, have room to attach a book rack—get smart *and* get fit at the same time!

- Set goals for yourself. If you're walking for 15 minutes a day now, for example, make it your goal to work up to 20 minutes next week. When you reach your goals, reward yourself!

- Chart your progress. Just like you keep track of your blood glucose or your food intake, keep an exercise log. This helps to reinforce the importance of exercise and allows you to track your progress.

- Don't feel guilty if you couldn't fit in your usual walk or trip to the gym. Focus on making the most of whatever activity you *are* doing that day. After all, housecleaning, stair climbing, raking, and gardening are all great ways to burn calories—and get those chores done at the same time!

- Help others while helping yourself. If you've been walking or jogging for exercise, consider doing a race or walking/running to raise money for a good cause, such as the American Diabetes Association.

Your Turn

Now it's your turn to recall some key points from this chapter. Let's see how you do!

1. List three benefits that exercise will give *you*:

   (1)_____

   (2)_____

   (3)_____

2. Hypoglycemia from exercise can be prevented by (circle all that apply):

   (1) Eating a snack before exercising
   (2) Taking more insulin
   (3) Taking less insulin
   (4) Drinking more water

3. List three things you will try to help you stay motivated to exercise:

   (1)_____

   (2)_____

   (3)_____

See APPENDIX A for the answers.

14

Dining Out

Joanne: I have to eat out for business at least four times week, but whenever I do, my blood sugars go sky high.

Dietitian: It sounds like maybe your portions are too large, or maybe you need some help with choosing more healthful items from the menu.

Joanne: You know, I think you're right. I've also gained about 10 pounds since starting my new job. Can you give me some hints on how I can eat out but still keep my weight and blood glucose under control?

Dietitian: Certainly. There's no reason that you can't enjoy eating away from home *and* stay healthy at the same time.

What's Next?

These days, eating away from home seems to be more of a reality than a treat for most people. Busy work and school schedules, "power lunches," and frequent travel often make cooking and eating at home difficult. Plus, with the wide variety of restaurants available, eating out is fun, not to mention sociable and quick. Who wants to spend an hour cooking dinner after a long day at work? All this eating away from home can wreak havoc for anyone, not just someone with diabetes. But it doesn't have to. Joanne learned that by making healthier menu choices she could eat out and still control her weight and blood glucose.

The Old and the New

Back in the early 1950s, only about 25 cents out of every food dollar was spent at a restaurant. Dining out was reserved for special occasions, such as birthdays and anniversaries. Today, eating out is still a treat for some of us, but it's an everyday thing for most of us. We spend almost 50 cents out of every dollar on restaurant meals. Consider some of these facts from the National Restaurant Association:

- In 1996, almost half of all adults (46%) ate at restaurants on any given day.
- In 1996, the typical person (age 8 or older) consumed an average of about four meals away from home each week.

- Almost 50 billion meals are eaten at restaurants or cafeterias each year.
- In 1995, the average annual household expenditure for food eaten away from home was about $1,700, or $680 per person.
- On a typical day in 1998, the restaurant industry has average sales exceeding $922 billion.

Here Are the Facts

Compare restaurant meals with those you prepare at home: portions are gargantuan; more than one course is served, starting with that basket of rolls on the table; many menu items are high in fat and calories; alcoholic beverages may be consumed; and the dessert menu is awfully tempting. Finally, the timing of restaurant meals may interfere with your usual diabetes medication or insulin schedule. Don't despair: There *are* ways to eat out *and* stay healthy. Believe it or not, you can choose healthful menu items in most restaurants and stay with your eating plan, while enjoying yourself at the same time.

Here's What You Can Do

A Smart Diner's Guide to Eating Out

1. **Refer to your meal plan.** Hopefully, by this point, you have met with a dietitian to establish some kind of an eating plan for yourself. This plan may involve using the food guide pyramid, the exchange system, or perhaps carbohydrate counting. Whatever you are

using, make sure you have a sense of how many servings, exchanges, or carbohydrate grams you need at each meal. Some people find that bringing a copy of their meal plan on a small card that they keep in their wallet helps when they eat out. Other people carry pocket-sized books that give carbohydrate and fat gram counts for various foods. A good book to try is *The American Diabetes Association Guide to Healthy Restaurant Eating* by Hope S. Warshaw.

2. **Learn serving sizes.** Okay, weighing and measuring foods isn't much fun. But you're not doomed to a lifetime of balancing a chicken breast on the scale or scooping pasta into a measuring cup. If you don't have a good sense of what a 4-ounce piece of meat or 1 cup of mashed potatoes looks like, take a few minutes the next time you're cooking to measure or weigh out your portions. (One hint: Always weigh and measure foods *after* cooking!) By measuring your foods a few times, you can start to train your eye to more accurately guesstimate portions. Check your technique periodically to make sure your portions haven't all of a sudden doubled in volume.

   Need some more help? Here's a trick you can use to gauge portions without having to lug your scale and measuring cups along to every restaurant. Visualize these everyday items to help make things a little easier:

   - a deck of playing cards = 3–4 ounces of meat
   - computer mouse = one medium potato
   - a teacup = 1/2 cup of ice cream or frozen yogurt
   - a light bulb = 1/2 cup of grapes
   - a baseball = 1 cup of fruit

- a tennis ball = one medium piece of fruit
- a walnut = 1 tablespoon of peanut butter

3. **Plan ahead.** This means several things. First of all, if you anticipate eating a somewhat fattier meal one evening, eat less fat that day at breakfast and lunch. Or if time permits, fit in some activity, such as a short walk around the block after your meal, to burn off some of those calories and keep blood glucose levels under better control. Second, don't forgo lunch or your afternoon snack (if you eat one) to "save room" for dinner. You'll be too hungry by the time your meal is served and may end up eating too much. Plus, if you take medication or insulin and you don't eat enough earlier in the day, you may end up with low blood glucose. Third, go ahead and call the restaurant ahead of time to inquire about the meals that are served and to ask if food can be prepared with less fat, sodium, etc.

4. **Take home leftovers.** With the size of restaurant meals these days, it's no wonder people end up leaving the restaurant groaning and loosening their belts. Don't feel you must force yourself to clean your plate of every morsel. Why not eat a reasonable portion, take the rest home, and have it for another meal the next day? Whether you call this "doggy-bagging" or bringing home leftovers, restaurants will happily accommodate your request to package up whatever you don't eat. If you're a lifelong member of the "Clean Plate Club"—as many people are—you might even ask the server to pack up half your meal in the kitchen before it's served to you. This way, you don't end up overeat-

ing *and* you've got a meal to go for tomorrow's lunch or supper.

5. **Share an entree with your dining companion.** Restaurant meals are certainly big enough for two people, so why not split a meal with your spouse or friend? If you like, order a salad, an extra potato or serving of rice, and maybe an extra vegetable. Plenty for everyone! Oh, and what about dessert? Once again, consider ordering one tiramisu or slice of pie for the table and having just a taste. Everyone will probably appreciate the calorie savings, while still enjoying that decadent dessert.

6. **Ask!** Be assertive with the server and politely, but firmly, let him or her know how you would like your entree prepared. For example, ask how many ounces the salmon weighs or for the dressing to be served on the side or for your scallops to be broiled without butter. Many restaurants have fresh fruit, low-fat salad dressings, or sugar-free syrups available, although these items may not be listed on the menu. Don't be afraid to speak up. You don't necessarily have to let anyone know that you have diabetes either. Remember that restaurants are service-oriented establishments, and they pride themselves not only on their food, but on how well you were served. After all, they want you to come back!

7. **Clear away the breadbasket.** A warm basket of freshly baked rolls or bread can hit the spot when you're waiting for your meal to be served. However, it may be so good that you eat more than you should. Help yourself to one if you like (remember to count this as a starch exchange or carbohydrate choice!), then request that the server remove the

basket from the table. Another suggestion is to order a bowl of broth-type soup or a tall glass of seltzer water to sip on. It will help fill you up and keep you from reaching for another piece of Italian bread.

8. **Order from the appetizer menu.** If you're looking for a light meal, glance over the appetizer section of the menu. You may be able to make a meal of two or three appetizers and bypass the heavier entrees altogether. Good choices might be shrimp cocktail, fruit cocktail, broth-based or tomato-based soups, raw vegetables, or a small salad. To round off the rest of your meal, order a baked potato, rice, or extra vegetables.

9. **Beware the buffets!** Buffets, or all-you-can-eat-style restaurants, can spell disaster for many diners. After all, who doesn't want to get his or her money's worth of food? Before you dig in, walk around the buffet to see what is offered. Note those food items that are lower in fat, such as vegetables, salads, poultry, and fish, and plan your meal around these items. Try one or two dishes that you don't usually eat for a treat. Don't feel that you must heap your plate full. You can always go back to try something else. Try not to let these situations throw you off your eating plan.

10. **Go easy with alcohol.** Many of us enjoy having a cocktail or glass of wine with our meals. However, the temptation to overindulge in good food and alcohol is frequently present. And alcohol, while fat-free, is a source of calories. People with diabetes need to be careful when drinking alcoholic beverages. It is important to understand how alcohol

itself can affect diabetes control. First, realize that alcohol is a drug, just like your diabetes medication or even aspirin. All drugs must pass through the liver to be detoxified and broken down. If you drink more alcohol than your liver can handle, the alcohol can affect your central nervous system and lead to symptoms of intoxication. Second, while most people with diabetes can drink alcohol in moderation, if your blood glucose levels are not in good control or if you have just completed exercise or vigorous activity, drinking alcohol can set you up for potentially severe hypoglycemia. The risk for hypoglycemia after having one or two drinks, even, is higher especially if you have not eaten for a while.

Use common sense if you decide to imbibe. Don't drink if you are pregnant; have a history of alcohol abuse; have heart, liver, or kidney disease; or have poorly controlled diabetes. *Always* eat something containing carbohydrate when you drink alcohol. Ideally, have the drink with your meal. If you're at a party, have a few pretzels or crackers. Don't substitute alcohol for carbohydrate choices or starch exchanges in your meal plan. If you're concerned about the calories in alcoholic drinks, substitute one drink (12 ounces of beer, 5 ounces of wine, or 1 1/2 ounces of liquor) for 2 fat exchanges.

11. **Deal with delays.** Frequently, eating out means that meals are served later than when you usually eat. If you take diabetes medications that don't work directly to lower your blood glucose, a delayed meal is not much of a concern. However, some diabetes medications, such as Micronase, Diabeta, and Glucotrol, can lower your blood glucose too much if

you don't eat at about the same times each day. If you take insulin, you also need to be aware of when your insulin is peaking and when you'll actually be eating. Talk to your doctor or dietitian about how best to deal with delayed meals.

Making Sense of Menus

Reading a restaurant menu can be a piece of cake if you know what to look for and what the various cooking terms mean. Most of us know that anything fried means high fat, but what about *sautéed, parmigiana,* or *au gratin?* If you're able to navigate your way around a menu, it will be much easier for you to choose healthful items and steer clear of excess fat and calories. When in doubt, ask your server to explain whatever is unclear, whether it's the actual definition of a term or how a particular dish is prepared. Here are some guidelines to get you started:

Go Ahead	Steer Clear
Baked (without butter)	Fried
Broiled (without butter)	Breaded
Roasted	Sautéed
Grilled	Creamed or creamy
Poached	Hollandaise
Steamed	Au gratin
Stir-fried	Scalloped/escalloped
Blackened	Buttered
Marinara	Alfredo
Cacciatore	Parmigiana
Au jus	Béarnaise

Commonly Asked Questions

I have to eat out at least three times a week because of my schedule. How can I control my portions? First, make sure you meet with a dietitian to work out a meal plan. Then, practice portion control at home, using measuring cups, spoons, and a scale. These tools will help train your eye for when you're eating out. Also, try relating your food portions to everyday objects, as in the examples above. Finally, remember it's okay to leave food on your plate. In fact, take it home for the next day.

If I drink a glass of beer, don't I have to substitute it for the starch at my meal? No, the beer is in addition to your meal. Alcohol has a blood-glucose-lowering effect, so don't eliminate your carbohydrate food at a meal. If your meal doesn't contain carbohydrate, you may have a low blood glucose later on. If you're concerned about the calories from beer, choose a light beer and eat less fat at your meal.

Sometimes the restaurant is slow serving my meal, but I've already taken my insulin. I'm concerned about hypoglycemia. What can I do? You could have a small snack while you're waiting, such as a roll or some crackers. Talk to your health care team about how to adjust for delayed meals, and ask about using Humalog insulin, which can be taken right before you eat.

Thinking that any seafood dish is low in fat, I ordered broiled scallops the other evening at a restaurant. When it was served, it was swimming in butter! What should I do next time? Don't always assume that broiled or baked foods are low in fat! The best thing to do is ask your server how a food is prepared before you order. If it sounds like too much fat is used in the cooking process, ask if the chef can prepare your dish with less fat, or at least a healthier fat such as olive oil.

Sometimes I end up overeating when I go to buffet-style restaurants. Is it okay to take a little more insulin after my meal to prevent my blood glucose from going too high? You shouldn't take more insulin—or more diabetes medication, for that matter—after your meal. Doing so could lead to low blood glucose later on. The best advice is to do some activity after you've eaten: go for a walk, do some housework, or hop on the exercise bike. This will help lower your blood glucose and burn calories at the same time.

Your Turn

Now it's your turn to recall some key points from this chapter. Let's see how you do!

1. List three things you can do to eat out more healthfully:

   (1)_____

   (2)_____

   (3)_____

2. A medium-sized potato is about the same size as a

   _____.

3. People with diabetes should never drink alcohol. True or false?

See APPENDIX A for the answers.

15

Food Cravings

Sarah: I generally do well with my eating plan, but every now and then I crave something sweet. Then I just give in and end up eating a whole box of cookies or a big candy bar.

Dietitian: Do you notice what brings on these cravings? Perhaps the time of day? Or do you think you're maybe depriving yourself too much of the foods you really like?

Sarah: Now that you mention it, I notice my cravings tend to pop up mid-afternoon at work, particularly when I'm feeling a little stressed and tired. Sometimes, too, I find myself eating ice cream right out of the container when I'm upset or anxious about something.

MYTH:

People with diabetes should never give in to food cravings.

Dietitian: Almost everyone experiences food cravings at some time or another. The key is learning how to deal with them before they get out of control and cause your blood sugars to get out of control.

What's Next?

Understanding and dealing with food cravings is complex. Researchers have developed many theories and ideas as to why people experience these cravings, and there's no agreement as to why they occur. What we do know about these mysterious and often frustrating cravings is that they happen because of a combination of physical and psychological factors. In other words, some of them may be "in your head," so to speak, but some arise because of occurrences in the body. Let's take a look at this intriguing aspect of nutrition.

The Old and the New

Do Our Bodies Know Best?

The idea that the body will crave or desire those nutrients it is lacking dates back to the 1930s and 1940s. The concept was called the "wisdom of the body." Back in the late 1920s, a pediatrician named Clara Davis published results of a study she conducted. In this study, three infants, ages 7 to 9 months, were offered a variety of healthy foods to choose from. The infants chose foods to comprise a healthy diet, all on their own, almost as if by instinct. Years later, in 1940, a psychologist named

Curt P. Richter published a study of a young boy who obsessively craved salt, often eating it straight from the salt shaker. When this boy was hospitalized and denied salt, he died. This boy had an adrenal gland disorder that caused his body to lose salt. The boy was eating salt literally to keep himself alive.

In more recent years, research by Judith Wurtman, a nutritional biochemist at Massachusetts Institute of Technology, has provided more evidence that, indeed, our bodies often give us signals when something is amiss in our diets. Dr. Wurtman has specifically studied people who are called "carbohydrate cravers." These people feel more energetic and less depressed after they eat carbohydrate-rich foods, such as bread or pasta. In fact, Dr. Wurtman has noticed that carbohydrate cravers are more likely to suffer from seasonal affective disorder (SAD), which is when people become more listless and depressed during the dark winter months. Eating more carbohydrate foods during that time of the year often helps people with SAD feel better. This mood improvement may have something to do with the release of a brain chemical called serotonin that seems to have a calming effect. Dr. Wurtman's research lends some weight to the idea that by craving carbohydrates the body is attempting to correct an imbalance, or deficiency.

Chemicals Causing Cravings?

Judith Wurtman's theory on carbohydrate cravers leads to the whole realm of how brain chemicals work to influence not only how and why we eat, but also our thoughts, feelings, and moods. The brain produces many substances, called neurochemicals, that can affect our appetite and food choices. *Serotonin* is one such neurochemical, called a neurotransmitter, that is produced from the amino acid tryptophan. Eating carbohydrate-containing foods triggers the entry of tryptophan into the brain, where it helps to form serotonin. Serotonin, in turn, has a calming, relaxing effect. The carbohydrate-serotonin theory suggests that an inadequate amount of carbohydrate in the diet causes serotonin levels to drop, thus leading to cravings for carbohydrate-rich foods, especially cakes, candies, and other sweets.

Not everyone fully agrees with this theory. Dr. Adam Drewnowski, director of the Human Nutrition Program at the University of Michigan, believes that people tend to crave fat rather than carbohydrate. Have you ever noticed what foods you end up eating when you have a craving? Chances are, if you have a sweet tooth, you'll eat "sweet fats," such as ice cream, cookies, or chocolate, instead of bread or even fat-free ice cream or cookies. Dr. Drewnowski claims it's the fat in these foods that we really want and that the added sugar just makes that food taste even better. The combination of fat and sugar releases endorphins in the brain, which are opiate-like chemicals that lift your mood and create an intense feeling of pleasure. Endorphins also act like the body's own natural painkillers. No wonder we find a piece of fudge or chocolate chip cookies more satisfying than a carrot stick!

But wait—there are even more neurochemicals that play a role in food cravings and appetite control. *Neuropeptide Y* (NPY) may actually trigger the desire for carbohydrates. NPY is released when the body is depleted of carbohydrates, for example, after strenuous exercise or a period of fasting. The inclination is to eat carbohydrate-rich foods in these situations, probably because of NPY. *Galanin,* another neurotransmitter, triggers the urge to eat high-fat foods, such as red meats, rich desserts, and creamy pasta sauces. Galanin levels tend to rise as the day goes on, when estrogen levels are high, and during weight loss. There is some evidence that obese people may have higher galanin levels than people of normal weight, which means that too much galanin or NPY secretion may eventually lead to weight gain.

To add insult to injury, stress plays a big role in food cravings. When we are under stress, our bodies release the "stress hormones" norepinephrine and corticosterone. These hormones can raise both NPY and galanin levels in the brain. This can lead to food cravings, overeating, and ultimately weight gain, if it happens often enough. Restrictive weight-loss diets don't help either. Low-calorie and even very-low-fat diets may disrupt the balance of these neurotransmitters, causing levels to actually increase, leading to overeating or even bingeing. In other words, over-restricting caloric intake may backfire and lead to weight gain. This can be even more frustrating if you have diabetes and are struggling to control your blood glucose.

Here Are the Facts

A craving can be formally defined as a consuming desire or a longing or yearning for something. All of us crave things, whether they be foods, a new car, or even companionship. Food cravings, in particular, commonly occur when you change your eating habits and start restricting or eliminating the foods that you like. After all, if you were told you could never eat chocolate chip cookies again—ever—what would you suddenly want? Chocolate chip cookies, of course! And nothing else would do.

Some people with diabetes feel this way frequently. Most people with diabetes are given a meal plan to follow to help control their blood glucose. A meal plan pretty much tells you when you can eat, how much you can eat, and what foods you can eat. Spontaneous eating seems out of the question, so if you're hungry at 5:00 P.M. but dinner is not supposed to be until 6:00, you either wait it out or end up grabbing something to eat—then feeling guilty.

People on stringent weight-loss diets often develop food cravings, and no wonder: they get hungry! How long can a meal of dry chicken and steamed broccoli satisfy you? Have you ever tried one of those fad diets where you eat just one or two foods for days at a time? How long did that last? Probably not too long. Were you dreaming of pizza or cake the whole time? Restrictive diets like these not only are unhealthy, but they often lead to intense cravings. This can result in bingeing, or overeating, often to the point where you may feel uncomfortable. On top of that, your blood glucose gets all out of whack.

We've learned more about cravings over the past two decades, and while they may always remain somewhat of a mystery, there are ways of understanding why they occur and how you can deal with them. There are even ways of fitting in your favorite foods on an occasional basis without wreaking havoc with your waistline and diabetes control.

Here's What You Can Do

If you have diabetes, you know that meal planning plays a major role in your diabetes control. Perhaps you haven't thought much about this, except to notice that now you need to eat meals on time or count carbohydrate grams. Did you ever stop and realize how much time you spend thinking about food? Diabetes can do this. Dietitians often hear people new to diabetes say, "I never used to eat candy before my diabetes, but now that's all I crave!" Another typical complaint often heard by dietitians is that people with diabetes who need to eat meals and snacks on time spend the day thinking constantly about food, to the point that they almost become obsessed!

Dieting, whether it be for weight reduction or blood glucose control, imposes its own rules and regulations on you. In a sense, you no longer have control over what, when, and how much you eat. It should come as no surprise then that you may not fare too well with the concept of dieting for long—and you're not alone. On top of following a "diet," you're also told that you must check your blood glucose levels daily, take your medication as directed, exercise, get your eyes examined yearly, and so on. The list is long. When you don't live up to all these expectations, you may either feel guilty or adopt a devil-may-care attitude because you can't be perfect 100% of the time. Many people end up bingeing on foods that aren't "on the meal plan."

If you can identify with some of these concepts and feel caught in a vicious cycle, it's important that you talk to your health care team. If you're experiencing feelings of deprivation surrounding foods, work with a dietitian who can show you how to fit favorite foods into your eating plan without throwing off your blood glucose control. In addition, it's particularly important to find a dietitian who will teach you that no foods are all "good" or all "bad"—*any* food can fit into a healthy eating plan. If you take insulin, talk to your health care team about learning how to adjust your insulin for the occasional extra carbohydrate you'd like to eat.

Make sure that you monitor your blood glucose when you splurge or try foods you haven't eaten for a while. Check your blood glucose before you eat a treat, then 1 1/2 to 2 hours later to see how that particular food affected your blood glucose. Share your results with your health care team if your results are high. They can help you think of ways to prevent high blood glucose after eating, whether it be through adjusting diabetes medication or insulin or increasing physical activity. Yes, you *can* have your cake and eat it too!

Taming Your Cravings

Everyone experiences cravings for foods. It is unrealistic to expect never to have a craving for something again. The key is to learn how to *manage* the craving before it results in something more drastic, such as an eating binge. As we said earlier, people with diabetes can be prone to problems with eating, depending on the advice they've been given by their health care team. After all, if your doctor has told you never to eat brownies again, you can be sure that brownies will be a constant visitor in your nightly dreams. It's better to learn how any food can be part of a healthful eating plan.

Let's discuss some techniques that may prove useful to you.

The first step is to learn the difference between hunger and appetite. Surprisingly, many people have no idea what it feels like to experience true physical hunger: stomach rumbling and pangs, headaches. People with diabetes are usually told they have to eat at regular times, whether they feel hungry or not; therefore, they may lose that sense of what being hungry means. Appetite, on the other hand, differs from hunger in that it may be triggered by certain emotions, places, or events (think of homemade stuffing on Thanksgiving). Hunger is more physiological, whereas appetite is more psychological. Not sure how to tell one from the other? It may take a while, but practice makes perfect. Ask yourself the following questions the next time you experience a craving. (And remember, it's okay to give yourself permission to feel *hungry* once in a while, as long as your blood glucose control is not affected).

- **When was the last time I ate?** If it's been more than 4 hours since your last meal, chances are your stomach is empty and is signaling you to eat something.
- **Is it hunger or appetite kicking in?** Again, if it's been a while since you last ate or you feel stomach pangs or feel light-headed, it's probably hunger. However, if you just ate lunch an hour ago, but you stepped into a candy store and the smell of chocolate hit you, you can say hello to your appetite.
- **Why do I want to eat right now?** Did you have a fight with your spouse or a bad day at work? Are you bored or lonely? Emotions are strong triggers for eating, especially uncontrollable eating.

- **What am I craving?** Whether you truly feel hunger or your appetite has been stimulated by a certain place or event, it's important to identify what it is you want. You may be surprised to find that what you really want is to soak in a nice, hot bath or to call up a good friend on the phone.

Ten Tips for Controlling Cravings

Now that you can distinguish between hunger and appetite, you're ready to tackle those cravings head on. Cravings will never go away for good, but you can take some measures to make sure they don't get out of control.

1. **Know your emotional triggers.** Emotions can be powerful triggers to eating. Stress, boredom, and loneliness can often lead to eating, especially "comfort" foods that seem soothing, at least initially. The problem, of course, with constantly eating to deal with emotions is that not only do you end up consuming far more calories than you need, but you really don't solve the problem. Instead of reaching for that package of cookies the next time you feel stressed, try another activity: go for a walk, call a friend, write a letter, drink a cup of hot tea, take a long, relaxing bath, or indulge in a hobby, such as knitting or wood carving. In fact, why not make a list of your own? That way, when emotions strike, you'll be prepared with an action plan. And if, despite all your efforts, your emotions seem to get the better of you, it may be wise to discuss this with your health care team, who may recommend you get professional help.

2. **Know your environmental triggers.** Your environment also plays a role in what, when, and how much you eat. For example, going to a party often leads to overindulging, simply because you're having fun. Are you a sports fan? If you went to any baseball or football games this past season, did you munch on hot dogs and peanuts? Sometimes your home environment can be the culprit. It's all too common for people to sit down to watch television after a hard day at work and end up snacking throughout the night. This can be a particularly tough habit to break, but it's not impossible. Here are some tips to try:

- Try not to keep high-fat, tempting goodies in the house.
- Ask family members to keep treats out of your sight.
- Eat only in one room, the kitchen or the dining room.

Finally, another helpful piece of advice is to start keeping a food journal. Write down everything you eat and drink and why. After a few days, you may see a trend emerging. At this point, think of an action plan to counteract this pattern.

3. **Wait those cravings out.** Cravings can vary in intensity. They may gradually build up, then peak in intensity, then fade away, almost like waves in the ocean. If you realize that cravings will come and go, you can prepare yourself. The next time that urge hits you, try waiting about 20 minutes for it to subside. Keep yourself busy doing something to take your mind off of it and it just might go away.

4. **Get going!** Not only does exercise take your mind off eating, it may help to suppress your appetite. In addition, studies show that aerobic exercise, such as walking or riding a bike, can stimulate the release of endorphins, chemicals in the brain that relieve pain and make us feel good.

5. **Separate eating from other events.** All too often, eating is combined with watching television or reading or even doing work at your desk. The process of eating should be treated as its own event. In other words, do nothing else when eating. You'll enjoy it more and you may be surprised that you end up eating a lot less. At the same time, the craving for high-fat snacks may subside once you limit eating in front of the television.

6. **Drink, drink, drink!** Nutrition experts all agree that an easy, effective way to curb cravings is to drink plenty of water. Liquids take up space in your stomach, thereby giving your appetite center in your brain the message "I'm full!" Aim to drink at least 8 to 10 glasses of water or other noncaloric fluids every day. You might even try sipping on hot tea or clear broth; some studies have shown that people who drink hot liquids eat less.

7. **Eat regular meals and snacks.** Okay, we said earlier that you should only eat when you feel hungry. But some people go all day without eating and end up with unbearable cravings and munchies at night. It's still important to eat at least three meals a day, with snacks in between. Not only does this help with your blood glucose control, but regular eating can actually help reduce the number of cravings you get and prevent overeating at night.

8. **Fit in fiber.** Fiber is an indigestible carbohydrate that has no nutritional value (see chapter 3) but does help increase satiety. Foods high in fiber include whole-grain breads, cereals, and crackers, as well fruits and vegetables. These foods take a while to chew, thereby slowing down your eating rate. And they take up room in your stomach, making you feel full sooner.

9. **Turn up the heat!** If you like hot, spicy foods, such as Mexican, Thai, or Szechuan dishes, go ahead and indulge. Spicy foods tend to satisfy your taste buds quicker than blander foods, so you usually eat less. You can put some heat in your dishes at home by adding chili powder, jalapeño peppers, or horse-radish. Another added benefit: Spicy foods speed up your metabolism.

10. **Count carbohydrates.** People who derive about 50 to 60% of their calories from complex-carbohydrate foods, such as potatoes, whole-grain bread, and pasta, tend to have fewer cravings for sweet carbohydrate foods, such as cookies and candy. Carbohydrate is the nutrient that has the most impact on blood glucose levels; therefore, people with diabetes need to control their carbohydrate intake. This does not mean, however, that you should be on a low-carbohydrate diet. What is helpful is to keep your carbohydrate intake consistent on a daily basis to keep blood glucose in good control and to keep those cravings away. Talk with your dietitian about learning how to count carbohydrates in your eating plan. For more information on carbohydrates, see chapters 2 and 3.

11. **Go ahead and give in.** What? You mean it's okay to indulge in that craving? Yes. It's important not to

deny yourself completely of the foods you love. Every now and then, especially when all other measures have failed, indulge a little and let yourself enjoy that food you've really been craving. Watch the portion and don't go overboard. It's better to have a small portion of what you *really* want than to fill up on foods that just don't satisfy that urge. Our motto: Everything in moderation.

Commonly Asked Questions

I seem to crave certain foods right when I get home from work. My cravings are worse when I've had a stressful day. Am I the only one who experiences this? No, you're not alone. Almost everyone has cravings, and they tend to be worse during stressful times. You may be eating in response to your stress or to fatigue or even just because you're hungry! Plan to have a small snack before you leave work to help prevent cravings.

I never used to eat sweets but now that I have diabetes, that's all I want to eat. Is this normal? Many people with diabetes experience sudden cravings for sweets, particularly when they are first diagnosed. Why this occurs isn't really known. However, the best thing to do is to discuss these cravings with a dietitian who can evaluate your eating plan and even help you fit in foods that you thought you "couldn't" eat (including sweets!).

Summary

Food plays an important role in everyone's lives. We eat for many reasons, some of which are simple, such as plain old hunger, and some of which are more complex, including emotions and environmental factors. Pay attention to your cravings and learn what causes you to eat. You may be surprised to find that the answer to dealing with cravings or uncontrolled eating is simple. If you need help, don't hesitate to talk with a therapist or counselor who specializes in the area of eating disorders. He or she can help you change how you think about and react to food and eating. Finally, remember that the act of eating is meant to be enjoyed and that you should not feel guilty if you indulge once in a while— even if you have diabetes! All foods can fit into anyone's eating plan.

Your Turn

Now it's your turn to recall some key points from this chapter. Let's see how you do!

1. Cravings can be triggered by strict dieting. True or false?
2. Only people with diabetes get cravings. True or false?
3. Waiting 20 minutes before "giving in" to your craving can help the craving subside. True or false?
4. List three triggers that set off your cravings:

   (1)_____

   (2)_____

   (3)_____

5. List three things you can do to help reduce or eliminate these triggers:

   (1)_____

   (2)_____

   (3)_____

6. Make a list of alternative activities you can do the next time a craving strikes. Post it on your refrigerator or bulletin board where you will easily see it.

See APPENDIX A for the answers.

16

Recipes

Lisa: Since I was diagnosed with diabetes 3 weeks ago, I haven't really known what I can eat. I packed up all my cookbooks and went out and bought some diabetic cookbooks, but to tell you the truth, some of the recipes don't look so good. And I'm not sure my family will like them, either.

Dietitian: There are actually many excellent cookbooks on the market geared toward people with diabetes. However, having diabetes doesn't mean you have to get rid of all your favorite recipes.

Lisa: But all my regular cookbooks have recipes that contain sugar and what seems like a lot of fat. I'm supposed to cut these things out of my diet.

MYTH:

People with diabetes have to throw out their favorite family recipes.

211

Dietitian: You don't have to *stop* eating sugar and fat. That's not realistic. But it is true that many cookbooks have recipes that are too high in fat. I can teach you how to modify your favorite recipes to be lower in both fat and sugar without sacrificing flavor.

Lisa: That sounds great! You mean I can still make my famous macaroni and cheese recipe for my family *and* myself?

Dietitian: You bet! Except now, it will be healthier for both you and your family.

The Old and the New

When was the last time you counted all the cookbooks on your bookshelf? If you're like many people, you probably have built up quite a collection over the years, ranging from Fannie Farmer to the latest low-fat, low-sodium, low-sugar diabetic cookbook. Today, there are literally thousands of cookbooks to be found in bookstores and cooking stores across the country. In fact, there are so many that you may find it overwhelming, especially if you have diabetes. Some cookbooks, of course, are better than others. At the end of this chapter, we'll recommend some cookbooks to help you out. However, the real purpose of this chapter is to teach you how to modify, or change, your existing recipes to make them a little lower in fat, sodium, and perhaps sugar.

Think back to when you found out you had diabetes. Most likely you were told you had to learn many different things, such as how to take insulin or medication, how to monitor your blood glucose, and how you should eat. Maybe you asked your dietitian or doctor for special "diabetic" recipes or cookbooks, thinking that you no longer could whip up your delicious food creations any more. Or if one of your family members was diagnosed with diabetes, perhaps you felt compelled to stop preparing many of the traditional family favorites and sacrifice flavor for dishes that didn't taste quite as good but were at least "diabetic."

Luckily, all that has changed today. The new nutrition guidelines for diabetes have changed the way people with diabetes can eat, and for the better. For example, sugar is no longer off-limits, since we now know that sugar is a carbohydrate just as starch is a carbohydrate (see chapters 2 and 3). Those infamous "diabetic diets" are now obsolete. There is no longer any such thing. Instead, you might be given an eating plan, or guide, to help you make better food choices. And while it's probably smart to keep an eye on your fat and sodium intake, you don't always have to eat bland low-fat, low-sodium foods all the time. Remember: Everything in moderation! People with diabetes should be eating the same as people without diabetes, incorporating nutrition principles from the USDA Food Guide Pyramid and the *Dietary Guidelines for Americans*. In other words, if you have diabetes, you do not need to eat any differently from the rest of your family, as long as the whole family eats healthy.

Here Are the Facts

These newer nutrition guidelines also mean something else when it comes to cooking: You do not necessarily need special diabetic cookbooks to cook and eat healthfully. Yes, there are plenty of wonderful cookbooks out there intended for people with diabetes. The good ones include healthy, yet tasty recipes that don't require a lot of special ingredients (including artificial sweeteners). They also provide nutritional information, such as carbohydrate and fat grams and exchanges, for each recipe. Another marker of a good diabetes cookbook is that the recipes should be geared toward *everyone* in the family, not just the person with diabetes. After all, who wants to prepare two different meals every night? Also, just because a cookbook contains healthful recipes doesn't always mean that they will taste good to *you*. Taste is very important—if you don't like a particular dish, most likely you'll never make it again.

If you glance through some of your older diabetes cookbooks, you'll notice that most of the emphasis is on cutting back or even eliminating sugar. Many of the diabetic recipes include artificial sweeteners or fructose as a substitute for sugar or honey. While you may still prefer to use artificial sweeteners when cooking, remember that it's not necessary to omit sugar from your recipes completely. In fact, depending on what you are cooking, sugar is sometimes even essential. Baked goods, such as quick breads, cookies, and cakes, require some sugar for leavening, texture, and flavor.

Once again, sugar is a carbohydrate, just like starch. Your blood glucose will rise if you eat too much of *any* kind of carbohydrate, even healthful foods such as breads, pasta, and fruit. Therefore, you don't have to avoid cooking or baking with sugar, but you *do* need to be careful of how much you eat of whatever you are cooking. And you may decide to reduce the sugar content in recipes anyway, simply because sugar adds empty calories.

The real culprit in the American diet is fat, not sugar. Americans get close to 40% of their calories from fat. The actual goal is less than 30% of calories from fat, with some health authorities even recommending no more than 20% of calories from fat. Too much dietary fat can lead to many health problems (see chapter 5). By reducing our fat intake and focusing on eating five or more servings of fruits and vegetables each day, we can make a difference in our health and hopefully prevent or delay the onset of major health problems. Most recipes can easily be adjusted to be lower in fat and therefore fit in with the dietary guidelines.

Sodium may be a concern for you, especially if you have high blood pressure or congestive heart failure. Just as with fat, high-sodium ingredients can be modified in any recipe. If you're concerned about flavor, rest assured that herbs and spices will substitute nicely for salt. Read the chapter on sodium (chapter 11) for more information.

Here's What You Can Do

We don't have room in this book to tell you everything you can do to modify your favorite recipes and cook more healthfully, but here are some suggestions for making substitutions that will get you started.

How to Substitute Ingredients

Thanks to the many lower-fat products available to us, such as fat-free or low-fat milk, cheeses, and margarine, it's relatively easy to make substitutions without dramatically affecting the final outcome (meaning taste and texture) of a recipe. However, some products work better than others. For example, it's not recommended to cook or bake with fat-free margarine because of its high water content. The same holds true for baking or heating fat-free cheese—you'll end up with a curdled lump of something closely resembling plastic! In addition, some people find that fat-free foods just don't taste good. If you don't like fat-free mayonnaise or fat-free sour cream, chances are you won't like the dishes in which you use these items.

Remember that not all fat is bad and that fat carries flavor. A little bit of fat is fine. You can often use the "real thing" in a recipe, but maybe use a little less of it. Or you might decide to trim fat at another meal that day to keep your fat calories down. Take the time to experiment with different ingredients to find what works and tastes best to you and your family.

Here are two general rules for baking with less fat and sugar:

- **Fat:** Use no more than 2 tablespoons of oil for every 1 cup of flour, and slightly increase one of the liquid ingredients to provide enough moistness.
- **Sugar:** Use no more than 1/4 cup of a nutritive sweetener (sugar, honey, molasses, corn syrup) for every 1 cup of flour. Reduce the amount of sweetener called for in a recipe by up to half the amount.

Ten Tips for Cooking with Less Fat

1. Use fat-free or low-fat milk in place of whole milk.

2. Use reduced-fat cheese or a smaller amount of strong-tasting cheese, such as Romano, sharp cheddar, or blue cheese.
3. Use egg whites or egg substitutes in place of whole eggs.
4. Use lean cuts of red meats, such as top round and tenderloin cuts, trimmed of fat.
5. Remove the skin from chicken and turkey after cooking.
6. Substitute ground turkey or chicken breast for some or all of the ground beef in a recipe.
7. Try "meatless" ground beef, usually made from soy, in place of ground beef.
8. Use canned tuna, salmon, and sardines packed in water, not oil.
9. Use low-fat or light mayonnaise, salad dressings, and margarine.
10. Marinate with low-fat salad dressing, flavored vinegar, or fruit juice in place of oil.

Sweeteners

Many recipes in diabetes cookbooks use nonnutritive, or artificial, sweeteners, such as saccharin, in place of some or all of the sugar in the regular recipe. The use of nonnutritive sweeteners can help reduce the calorie content of the recipe as well as the carbohydrate content somewhat; however, remember that there will still be carbohydrate in the dish if it contains flour, oatmeal, fruit, etc. You need to account for this carbohydrate in your meal plan.

The use of nonnutritive sweeteners in baking and cooking is often a matter of individual preference. Now that you know that sugar is no longer off-limits and that you can reduce the sugar content in recipes by half, you may decide not to use nonnutritive sweeteners at all. Some people object to using "chemicals," while others simply do not like how they taste. Decide what's best for you. If you choose to use a nonnutritive sweetener, do not automatically eliminate the sugar in the recipe. Sugar is there not only to provide sweetness, but also to provide volume, moistness, tenderness, and color. Without sugar, cakes, muffins, and quick breads would be flat, dry, and tough. Nonnutritive sweeteners don't have the same properties as sugar. A good rule of thumb is to substitute *half* of the sugar called for with a nonnutritive sweetener.

There are four types of sweeteners on the market available for cooking and baking: saccharin, aspartame, acesulfame K, and sucralose. The most common brand names, respectively, include Sweet'n Low, Equal, Sweet One, and Splenda, although there are others. All sweeteners list directions on the box for how to substitute for sugar. Remember, too, that sweeteners are *very* sweet, so you use much less of them than you would sugar. (See chapter 6.) Here's a quick reference to get you started:

For 1/4 cup sugar use one of the following:
- 6 packets of aspartame
- 6 packets of saccharin
- 3 packets of acesulfame K
- 1/4 cup sucralose

(By the way, using one of these sweeteners in place of 1/4 cup sugar saves 170 calories and 60 grams of carbohydrate. And if you are baking with sweeteners, you may be wise to choose saccharin, acesulfame K, or sucralose instead of aspartame; under high temperatures, aspartame may break down and impart a slightly bitter aftertaste.)

What about other sweeteners, such as honey, molasses, fructose, sugar cane juice, or fruit juice? The bottom line is that sugar is sugar, no matter what the form. If you prefer to use these sweeteners because they are less refined, that's fine, but they still contain calories *and* carbohydrate. In addition, some recipes don't work well if you use, for example, honey in place of sugar. If you want to go ahead with a substitution such as this, first read the recipe or cookbook for special instructions. If those aren't available, pretend you're a chemist and experiment! You'll never know until you try.

One final word about using less sugar in recipes: If you're concerned that your banana bread or pumpkin pie just won't taste the same without as much sugar, make sure you add flavorful spices such as cinnamon, nutmeg, or ginger. Extracts, too, can bring out the sweetness in a food. Try vanilla, almond, or any flavor extract.

Salt and Sodium

Many people need to reduce their sodium and salt intake, especially if they have high blood pressure. Some people choose to cut back simply to stay healthy. Salt, like fat, provides flavor. Therefore, you may be somewhat reluctant to eliminate salt or other high-sodium ingredients from a recipe for fear the outcome will taste bland and boring. The good news is that you probably have in your cupboard or pantry a whole array of flavorful herbs and spices that work just as well, if not better, than your salt shaker. You can even concoct your own herb and spice blends or refer to cookbooks for ideas. Or to make things easier, purchase premade herb and seasoning blends right in your grocery store.

Recommended Cookbooks

There is a vast array of cookbooks on the market. Many of these cookbooks are excellent; unfortunately, we don't have room here to list them all. Below is a list of cookbooks that we've chosen to help you in your quest to cook and eat more healthfully. Not all of these are geared toward diabetes, either. Hopefully, after reading this chapter, you feel more confident in making modifications and substitutions on your own. And remember, you don't have to take your old cookbooks to the library book sale: modify those recipes that you like.

The Joslin Diabetes Gourmet Cookbook by Bonnie Sanders Polin, PhD, and Frances Towner Giedt with the Nutrition Services Staff at the Joslin Diabetes Center, Bantam, 1993

The Joslin Diabetes Quick and Easy Cookbook by Frances T. Giedt and Bonnie S. Polin, PhD, with the Nutrition Services Staff at the Joslin Diabetes Center, Fireside/Simon & Schuster, 1998

The Complete Quick & Hearty Diabetic Cookbook by the American Diabetes Association, 1998

Diabetic Meals in 30 Minutes—Or Less! by Robyn Webb, American Diabetes Association, 1996

Commonly Asked Questions

How can I bake cakes and cookies with less sugar? Try reducing the sugar content in recipes by one-half. Slightly increase one of the liquid ingredients in the recipe to give moistness.

I'm tired of baked chicken. What other healthy way can I prepare it? Consider buying a wok and start stir-frying! It's quick, easy, and healthful. Or get a Crock-Pot and make a chicken stew that will simmer all day and be ready in time for dinner. Finally, marinate chicken breasts in low-fat salad dressing or a small amount of oil and balsamic vinegar, then broil, grill, or bake.

I occasionally cook with bacon, but I know how fatty it is. Any good substitutes? Try turkey bacon. It contains half the fat of regular bacon. Other good choices are Canadian bacon, which is much leaner than regular bacon, or vegetarian "bacon," which is usually made from soybeans.

I have a recipe for a decadent cheesecake that I like to make for my family, but I know how high in fat it is. Is there any way I can make it lower in fat? It contains cream cheese, sour cream, and eggs. You can certainly make it lower in fat by altering a few ingredients. First, try low-fat cream cheese. Second, use light sour cream. And third, use egg whites or an egg substitute in place of the eggs. There will still be some fat in this cheesecake but a whole lot less!

Your Turn

Now it's your turn to recall some key points from this chapter. Let's see how you do!

1. Since you have diabetes, you must eliminate all the sugar in your recipes. True or false?
2. You can eat all you want of foods made with nonnutritive sweeteners. True or false?
3. Try your hand at modifying the recipe below. Think about how you can reduce both the fat and sodium content of this recipe.

Mexicali Casserole

---

2 large onions, chopped	2 1-lb cans tomatoes and juice
1 cup chopped bacon	2 1-lb cans corn, drained
2 lbs ground beef	3 cups yellow cornmeal
2 lbs ground pork	3 cups whole milk
2 tablespoons salt	4 eggs, well beaten
2 tablespoons chili powder	1 cup pitted black olives
2 cloves garlic	

Saute onions and bacon until tender. Add ground beef, pork, salt, chili powder, and garlic and stir. Add in tomatoes and their juice and the corn. Cook for 5 minutes. Next, add cornmeal, milk, beaten eggs, and olives. Turn into a large casserole dish or baking pan. Bake at 300 degrees for 1 1/2 hours. Serves 20.

See APPENDIX A for the answers.

"Your Turn" Answer Key

Chapter 1, page 12

1. medical nutrition therapy
2. true
3. 6 or more (Grains, Beans, and Starchy Vegetables)
   3–5 (Vegetables)
   2–4 (Fruits)
   2–3 (Milk)
   2–3 (Meat and Others)
4. true

Chapter 2, pages 25 and 26

1. sugar
2. true
3. sugar, starch, fiber
4. fruits, vegetables, milk

5. candy, regular soda (and other sweets)
6. true

Chapter 3, page 38
1. true
2. fiber (or dietary fiber)
3. starch, fiber
4. true

Chapter 4, page 54
1. false
2. chicken, fish, eggs (and other meats or dairy products)
3. kidney beans, peanut butter, tofu (and other beans or nuts)
4. name a vegetarian meal

Chapter 5, page 68
1. triglycerides
2. saturated
3. fat, protein
4. protects our major organs; prevents dry skin; maintains our body temperature; stores vitamins A, D, E, and K; intensifies the taste of foods

Chapter 6, pages 79 and 80
1. true
2. 5, 20, 3 or 4
3. caloric, noncaloric
4. aspartame
5. answers will depend on the foods you choose

Chapter 7, page 92
1. false
2. false
3. 100, 60, 10
4. true

Chapter 8, page 107

1. true
2. serving size
3. five
4. three

Chapter 9, page 122

1. true
2. false
3. false
4. reduce portions, start exercising, eat less fat (and others)
5. answers will be up to you

Chapter 10, page 138

1. false
2. true
3. vitamin C, vitamin E, or beta-carotene
4. whole-grain breads or cereals, legumes, nuts, bananas, or green leafy vegetables (pick any two)

Chapter 11, page 153

1. 2,400
2. false
3. false
4. don't use the salt shaker, eat fresh or frozen vegetables instead of canned, use fewer
5. high-sodium condiments (and others)

Chapter 12, pages 165 and 166

1. exercise
2. appetite, meals
3. grazing, permission to skip a meal, eating junk food, a cause of weight gain, keeping junk foods in the house, being hungry (pick any three)
4. false

Chapter 13, page 181
1. better blood glucose control, weight control, healthier heart (and others)
2. eating a snack before exercising, taking less insulin
3. start out gradually, exercise with a friend, keep track of progress (and others)

Chapter 14, pages 193 and 194
1. plan ahead, take home leftovers, limit alcohol (and others)
2. computer mouse
3. false

Chapter 15, pages 209 and 210
1. true
2. false
3. true
4. feeling bored, waiting too long to eat, being told you can't eat a certain food (and others)
5. do another activity, such as exercising; don't keep tempting foods around; don't eat when watching TV (and others)
6. call a friend, go for a walk, clean the house, keep a journal (and many others)

Chapter 16, page 222
1. false
2. false
3. suggestions: use ground turkey in place of ground beef/pork; use turkey bacon; reduce amount of salt used; use skim milk in place of whole milk; use egg whites in place of eggs

Dietitians and Diabetes Educators

What Is a Registered Dietitian?

You may not think twice about the difference between a nutritionist and a dietitian. But there is a difference. A person can claim to be a nutritionist whether he or she has had training in nutrition or not. A registered dietitian, however, is required to have a bachelor's degree from an accredited college or university, to have completed specific coursework in nutrition and nutrition-related sciences, to have completed an internship at an accredited institution, and to have passed a national exam administered by the American Dietetic Association. In addition, every 5 years, this person must acquire 75 hours of continuing education to stay registered. This ensures that the dietitian is up-to-date with the latest developments and research in the field of nutrition. A registered dietitian will have the credentials "RD" after his or her name, which means the person has completed academic and experience requirements established by the Commission on Dietetic Registration, an agency of the American Dietetic Association.

What Does a Registered Dietitian Do?

A registered dietitian is uniquely qualified to establish an eating plan for you that will meet your requirements and your goals. Your doctor or health care team may suggest you see a dietitian for certain conditions or situations, including:

- diabetes
- high cholesterol or high triglycerides
- high blood pressure
- overweight or obesity
- gastrointestinal disorders
- pregnancy
- unexplained weight loss
- lack of energy
- nutrient deficiency

A dietitian will take into consideration your requirements and food preferences. He or she will work with you to develop an individualized plan that provides you with a variety of foods and adequate nutrients.

Where Can I Find a Registered Dietitian?

You can find a registered dietitian in your area by calling your local hospital or by calling The American Dietetic

Association's Nationwide Nutrition Network at 1-800-366-1655. In addition, each state has a dietetic association that can provide you with referrals to dietitians near your home. You can even access The American Dietetic Association on the Internet at *www.eatright.org* for further information.

What Is a Diabetes Educator?

If you have diabetes, the person who taught you how to check your blood glucose or the person who developed a meal plan for you may have been a diabetes educator. A diabetes educator is a health professional—a nurse, a dietitian, an exercise physiologist, a social worker, even a doctor—who specializes in treating and educating people with diabetes. You can find diabetes educators working in hospitals, outpatient clinics, doctors' offices, and nursing homes.

A diabetes educator is identified by the credentials "CDE," which stand for certified diabetes educator. To become a CDE, a health professional must first work in the field of diabetes care for a specific number of hours. Once that number of hours has been reached, the person takes a national qualifying exam to become certified. Being a CDE entitles the health professional to educate and treat people with diabetes. For example, a CDE can help you adjust your insulin, establish an insulin-to-carbohydrate ratio, or learn to inject insulin. Every 5 years, a diabetes educator who is a CDE must take the exam again to make sure he or she is aware of new developments and treatments in the area of diabetes care.

What Does a Diabetes Educator Do?

Diabetes educators can teach you the skills you need to manage your diabetes. The following types of educators may be part of your diabetes care team:

- **Nurse educator (RN, CDE):** Nurse educators can help you understand how your diabetes medication or insulin works. They may teach you how to draw up insulin and give yourself an injection, or they may teach you how to use a blood glucose meter. Nurse educators can also show you how to deal with special situations, such as sickness, pregnancy, or travel.
- **Registered dietitian (RD, CDE):** A dietitian who is a diabetes educator has advanced knowledge in meal planning for people with diabetes. For example, maybe you'd like to learn carbohydrate counting or how to eat vegetarian meals while following a meal plan. Dietitians can also help people with diabetes who have special needs, such as children, adolescents, overweight adults, and people with kidney problems.
- **Exercise physiologist:** An exercise physiologist has also had specific training to help people with diabetes learn how to exercise safely. Many people with diabetes have other health concerns, such as heart disease, neuropathy, or retinopathy. An exercise physiologist understands these conditions and can prescribe a program that fits a person's needs.
- **Mental health provider:** A mental health provider, such as a social worker or psychologist, can be indispensable in providing support to you and your family. Having diabetes means that you face daily

challenges that can often be overwhelming to you and your loved ones. Meeting with a mental health provider gives you a chance to talk about your concerns and fears about having diabetes, particularly if you are feeling that your diabetes is out of control. A mental health provider can also help you adjust to changes in your life, such as a new job or getting married, without affecting your diabetes self-care.

Certified diabetes educators are members of the American Association of Diabetes Educators (AADE). You can find a diabetes educator by contacting AADE at (312) 424-2426 or on the Internet at *www.aadenet.org*. You can also find a recognized diabetes education program in your area by contacting the American Diabetes Association at 1-800-DIABETES or on the Internet at *www.diabetes.org*.

Index

Abdominal fat, 112
Acceptable daily intake (ADI), for
    sweeteners, 73–74
Acesulfame K (acesulfame
    potassium), 70, 74, 219
Adolescents, supplements needed by,
    134
Aerobic exercise, 172–173
Alcoholic beverages
    empty calories in, 5
    only in moderation, 5
    in restaurant eating, 189–190
    serving size, 9
American Association of Diabetes
    Educators (AADE), 227
American diet, 4
American Dietetic Association, The,
    6, 27, 84, 224–225
American Heart Association, 140,
    148
Amino acids, 42
Animal products, 10, 48
    protein in, 45–46
Antioxidants, 128–131, 136
Appetite. *See also* Food cravings
    controlling, 157
    different from hunger, 203
    and emotional factors, 121,
        203–204
    satisfying, 10, 83, 89–90

    suppressed by exercise, 206
Arteries, clogged, 64
Aspartame, 70, 73, 219

Baking. *See also* Recipes
    using whole-grain flours in, 36
Beans, serving size, 8
Blood glucose levels, 11
    controlling, 4, 16, 64, 78–79, 131
    and eating out, 190–191
    self-monitoring, 15, 202
Blood pressure. *See also* High blood
    pressure
    monitoring, 148
    primer on, 144–148
Body mass index (BMI), 113–115.
    See also Weight
Breads
    in restaurant eating, 188–189
    whole-grain, 10

Calcium supplements, 136
Calories. *See also* Empty calories
    enough for keeping reasonable
        weight, 4
    from fat, 64
    understanding, 116–117
Carbohydrate counting, 81–92, 207
    budgeting your daily allowance, 88
    versus exchange lists, 87–88

Family
    asking for help, 179
    educating, 11
Fat, abdominal, 112
Fats in blood, reaching optimal levels
        of, 4
Fats in food, 55–68
    choosing, 5
    cutting down on, 10, 37,
        117–118, 215
    defined, 58–59
    focusing on first, 117
    foods containing, 61–62
    "good" and "bad," 58–59
    need for, 62–63
    negotiating, 91
    serving size, 9, 64
    substituting in recipes, 215–217,
        221–222
    total on food labels, 103
"Fewer," claims stating, 98–99
Fiber, 10, 17, 27–38
    added, 101
    increasing intake of, 35–36, 118,
        207
    need for, 33
    soluble and insoluble, 32–33
Fish, serving size, 9
Food and Drug Administration
        (FDA), 74, 97
Food cravings, 195–210
    defined, 199–200
    emotional triggers, 204
    environmental triggers, 205
    giving in to, 207–208
    taming, 202–208
    theories about, 196–199
Food labels. See Label reading
Foods
    restricted, 11
    serving sizes, 8–9
    variety in, 5, 10
"Free," claims stating, 98
Fructose, 17–18, 70

Fruits, 5
    serving size, 8, 36

Galactose, 17–18
Galanin, 199
"Generally Recognized as Safe"
        (GRAS) ingredients, 74
Glucose, 17–18. See also Blood
        glucose levels
    carrying source of, 176
"Good source," claims stating, 99
Grain products, 5
    serving size, 5, 36
Guidelines, 11, 14
    for activity, 169
    for exercise, 172
    for reading menus, 191–193
    for smart snacking, 159–161,
        205

HDL cholesterol, 60
Health, improving overall, 4
Health claims, 97–98
Heart disease
    reducing risk of, 35, 64, 129–130,
        132
    risk factors for, 66, 112, 115
High blood pressure, reducing risk
        of, 64, 112, 140–148, 152
"High in," claims stating, 99
Hunger, 161, 203. See also Food
        cravings
Hydrogenated oils, 67
Hydrogenated starch hydrolysates
        (HSH), 76
Hyperglycemia, and physical activity,
        177–178
Hyperlipidemia, 59, 65
Hypoglycemia
    and alcoholic beverages, 190
    and restaurant eating, 192
    treating safely, 78–79, 175–178,
        181